VISCERAL: ESSAYS ON ILLNESS NOT AS METAPHOR

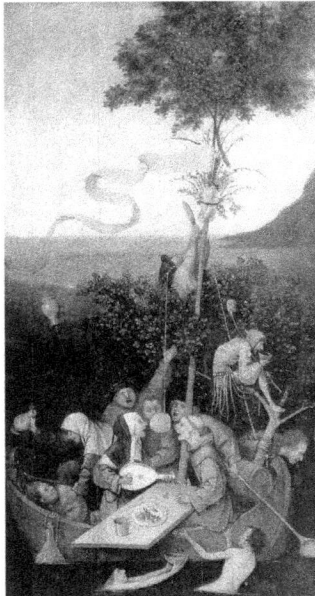

Fig. 1. Hieronymus Bosch, Ship of Fools (1490–1500)

Visceral

Essays on Illness Not as Metaphor

* * *

Maia Dolphin-Krute

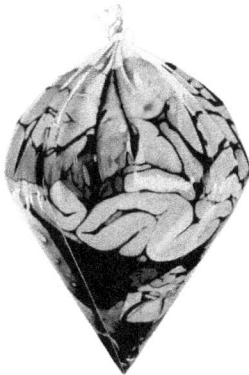

Brainstorm Books
Santa Barbara, California

brainstorm books

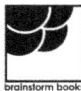

First published in 2017 by Brainstorm Books
An imprint of punctum books, Earth, Milky Way
www.punctumbooks.com

ISBN-13: 978-1-947447-26-4 (print)
ISBN-13: 978-1-947447-27-1 (ePDF)

LCCN: 2017956831
Library of Congress Cataloging Data is available from the Library of Congress

Editorial team: Karla Bernardo, Julie Carlson, Rebecca Elster, Kristen McCants, and Natalie Wong
Book design: Kristen McCants
Cover design: Karla Bernardo
Cover artwork (front): Simon Goinard, "Within," [no date]
Cover artwork (back): Fábio Magalhães, "Sem Título" (Série Retratos Íntimos), 2013

Contents

Acknowledgments

This book was written over several months in 2015 during which I was visiting, calling, or having procedures done at Brigham and Women's Hospital almost every other week. As stressful as that may have been, I am deeply thankful to Brigham and Women's for providing an unparalleled level of care, and especially to Dr. Peter Banks — it remains the only hospital I have ever been in without yelling at a single staff member (apologies to Smilow Cancer Care Center at Yale). I am also very thankful to Eileen Joy and Chris Piuma at punctum books for their support of this project, and to *Full-Stop* and Meagan Day, who first published the essay "Daily Survivor #1." And as always, none of this could have happened without the unending support, care, and patience of the Dolphins, the Krutes, and the Dolphin-Krutes, and of Jesse Kenas Collins, a daily survivor-caregiver in his own right.

Smilow

I am standing in a fluorescent-lit hallway at 6:45AM. It is actually, probably, closer to 7:00AM; 6:45 was when I got here. Behind me are double glass doors, shut, heavy. The rest of the corridor is in front of me, turning off to the right at a midway point, but what's there I can't see. It would be the kind of opening for an elevator bank. There are elevators behind me, too, if you made a right from the glass doors instead of pushing them open into an also fluorescent-lit office. Bathrooms also. Bathrooms with heavy doors but faulty locks, bathrooms I have already been in, twice, in fifteen minutes, first out of necessity and then to wash my face to keep from or stop crying. I am in the Shapiro Cardiovascular Center at 6:45 in the morning. My insurance company has just declined to cover a CT scan I came here to get. Although the doors are heavy, now, afterwards, I wonder whether anyone inside the imaging center heard me on the phone, when I called my father to (begin to) sort this out, when I started (or tried to keep from) crying, when I cursed in a loud or maybe not that loud voice. It was hard to tell, because until 6:45 on this Monday, I had never been down here, on level 2, of the Shapiro Cardiovascular Center at Brigham and Women's Hospital.

Emblem

In his now classic work, *A Pattern Language,* architect Christopher Alexander lays out, in three volumes, a method of planning for and building a town and all of the many kinds of buildings within it. The pattern is really more of a series, of pieces and structures from

"Architectural Valleys" and "Building Thoroughfare" to "Floor Surface" and "Filtered Light," which can be chosen from and fitted together depending on the needs of the project at hand. The pattern includes, or describes, not only buildings but what goes on in them: infrastructure. For piece 147, "Small Services Without Red Tape," Alexander describes the way that bureaucracy, whether governmental or private, should function so as to remain as accessible as possible. That is, in his words, to remain human, and not become impersonally bureaucratic. To do this, "no service should have more than 12 persons total…12 seems to be the largest number of people that can sit down in a face to face discussion."[1] Though he doesn't say why it seems like this, only one reason comes to mind: When is a group of 12 people in a face-to-face discussion ever anything but a jury?

Nesson

I've never been down here, a basement if it weren't a hallway, if there weren't even other levels below L2, because usually I go to the Richard H. Nesson Ambulatory Care Center at Brigham and Women's Hospital. There, they have rows of snake plants and zamiifolia plants dividing space in the front entrance; Shapiro has only snake plants. Nesson is also fluorescently lit, though there are windows in the waiting room of the doctor I go there to see. The blinds are usually partially drawn. They do not stock magazines. The bathroom in the hallway outside the (also heavy but wooden) doors of the practice also has a faulty lock. There is a number you can text to report facilities complaints like this (I don't).

I have not been to Nesson since August. When I was at Shapiro, it was the beginning of September. I have not been to Shapiro again since then, because my insurance company has continued to deny coverage for the CT scan or anything else that takes place in Shapiro or Nesson or other Brigham and Women's buildings. Is this

---

1   Christopher Alexander, Sara Ishikawa, Murray Silverstein, Max Jacobson, Ingrid Fiksdahl-King, and Shlomo Angel, *A Pattern Language: Towns, Buildings, Construction* (New York: Oxford University Press, 1977), 405.

continued denial one by a jury? Would it be better, more understandable (more human), if it were?

Smilow

When I am in places like Shapiro and Nesson or the Smilow Cancer Care Center at Yale New Haven Hospital, where I have also been a patient, are these places really like other buildings? Or, more specifically, is being in these places more like being in a building or more like being with people? Are Nesson and Shapiro and Smilow only physical spaces or people who have shaped physical spaces? How do these people shape one's experience of a place?

After visits to Smilow Cancer Care Center, my mother and I would go to a nearby Ikea, which I loved, because how nice to walk through fluorescent-lit spaces that tell you where to go so specifically they even have arrows on the floor. I don't know if Christopher Alexander would approve or not.

Emblem

Yesterday, almost a month after the first and only time I was in the Shapiro Cardiovascular Center, I went to the website of Emblem Health, my insurance company. It's the only place of theirs that one can visit. Or, seeing as how they do, actually, run several community health centers in and around New York, the website is the only place one who is distinctly out-of-network and not there in person can go. The website features a blog called "Who's Caring For You?" Good question. I'd like to ask them. I'd like to ask them in an email, since I have no in-person options, an email that would be more like a poem. Both because a poem is neither a threat nor a complaint, nothing that could be deserving of retaliation, nor is it something that could be wholly understood or answered. "Who's Caring For You?"

Shapiro

Are networks always about what is within and outside of them? Like collections, in a way, because the moment something is called a collection what becomes most apparent are all of the things still to collect. Networks provide a surface over this absence, though, a net, really, that seems all encompassing. Community health centers. Or, if not all-encompassing, familial, like how Carl J. and Ruth Shapiro's son-in-law is the Chief of Surgery at Brigham and Women's Hospital. I wonder how Shapiro's endowment of the building affects his son-in-law's presence in its surgical suites, how different this presence is from my own.

His other son-in-law is a broker. Investment is, actually, the source of most of Shapiro's wealth. Like the $25 million donation that created the Carl J. and Ruth Shapiro Cardiovascular Center. Which was $600 million less than the settlement Shapiro reached with the United States government after his potentially complicit involvement in Bernie Madoff's Ponzi scheme came to light.[2]

Networks become gothic.

Emblem

The fluorescent-lit hallways at both Shapiro and Nesson are striking on multiple levels. Not only because of their overall dimness, their basement feel, but because of how at odds with certain tenets of architecture this fluorescence is. Namely the relationship between light and buildings that developed during the Age of Reason; the Enlightenment, literally. Architecture became a way of letting in the light, a way to embody a clearing out and lighting up of the dark spaces of human minds. Fluorescent lights do not make things particularly clear.

I am drawn instead to the bright white margins and naturally lit photographs of "Who's Caring For You?" The bright white is at odds with the very gothic nature of the Emblem Health HIP network and the buildings it takes place (and doesn't take place) in. "Gothic" both in the sense of haunted and as in gothic architecture and the way that is marked in particular by an excess of ornamentation.

---

2   Beth Healy and Todd Wallack, "Madoff Client to Return $625 Million," *The Boston Globe,* December 8, 2010, http://archive.boston.com/yourtown/boston/roxbury/articles/2010/12/08/madoff_client_settles_with_us_for_625m/.

"Emblem" is too easy. It would be too easy to read "Emblem" within ornamentation, as one of the many signs of faceless bureaucrats, covered over by the ornamentation bureaucracy provides. Emblematic.

Instead, what I am reminded of is the common technique of being taught to draw by using one's body to measure the distance between two things or their size. You hold your hands up, with one eye closed, superimposing your thumb or arm on the scene, imaginary marks being made in your mind's eye, on your body, marks that can then be transferred to those same objects on your paper. It's a remarkably accurate process. It's remarkably accurate the way the body can be used as a measuring device more generally: How many steps between elevator, bathroom and heavy glass doors? How long did I look at "Who's Caring for You?" before curiosity became the rage unique to bureaucratic anger? How far out-of-network, out of Emblem Health HIP (out of being emblematic, out of health) am I, and how can this distance be recorded through the absences in my body? Will my insurance company consider certain forms of entropy as a kind of co-pay? The unabashed yearning at the heart of this out-of-network state is gothic.

Of course the insurance company won't really take my body's losses as a kind of payment. Some states do have a form of medical error litigation based on the idea of a "lost chance;" as in, if error hadn't prevented your timely diagnosis, you would have had the chance to live longer or to just not die altogether. "Have had" being the key words here. "Have had," as in having had the pains and various symptoms I'm (not) currently being tested for, for anywhere from four months to four years, depending on the specific symptom, at what point (if any) were chances lost? If an illness is chronic do I still get any chances? S. Lochlann Jain details further paradoxes at the heart of medical malpractice litigation: "It is truly ironic that, while basing large fees on the inherent value of life, the medical industry with its doctors, lawyers and administrators, have been able at the same time to lobby for caps on damage awards in most states, stunting that same valuation."[3]

---

3   Sarah Lochlann Jain, *Malignant: How Cancer Becomes Us* (Berkeley, CA: University of California Press, 2013), 101.

I suppose what I really meant, earlier, about Michael Zinner (Carl J. Shapiro's son-in-law) and my presences in the Brigham and Women surgical suites was that I currently owe the hospital $1,600 for a surgery I had several months ago (because my insurance chose to pay only $700 of a $2,300 bill) and how, exactly, does this money (that ultimately my father paid) stand in relation to Zinner's father-in-law's money? What do the amounts or responsibilities for payment say about the positions of our bodies in the hospital?

Lochlann goes on to write that, in medical malpractice cases, "juries disproportionately favor physicians."[4] Maybe this is why "Small Services With No Red Tape" function best with only 12 people: Juries come to a consensus about what is important to uphold. Why is it that 12 is the example given and not, say, a classroom, a larger group of people; a group, though, who can leave the room before a consensus is reached?

Smilow

Much as medical malpractice lawsuits are caught between different, opposing ways of valuing life, so too are buildings caught between different sets of values. Although it's not, actually, that life and the value of it set the opposition in medical malpractice cases, it's who is paying for that life.

Architecture is seen as existing within "a sanctified and aestheticized cultural sphere of value (understood as inspiration, creation, taste, test of time, intrinsic and transcendental value) and, on the other [hand], within an economic sphere of value (calculation, references, costs, benefits, prices and utility."[5] In some settings these values coalesce beautifully, places that are (or sell) affordable, timeless (but also current) good design and make that design easy to navigate. Ikea. Hospital architecture is both an intensification of the distinction between these sets of values and completely exempt from critique under most of them, because hospitals are pure utility; they are meant to do a thing and do it well, and keep removed from overt reminder that a large part of the thing it does is make

4 Jain, *Malignant,* 101.
5 Stephen Cairns and Jane Jacobs, *Buildings Must Die: A Perverse View of Architecture* (Cambridge, MA: MIT Press, 2014), 49.

you pay for your body. Keep it from overt reminder through things like water features (in the foyer of Smilow Cancer Care Center) and those rows of zamiifolia plants and snake plants, which I usually notice more than I notice how much I am paying (or my family or my father's employer or Emblem Health HIP is paying) for my body, except in moments when I am told that no one will be paying. "Who's Caring For You?"

Maybe it feels that hospital architecture is in some ways exempt from the values of other forms of architecture because it is Carl J. Shapiro's name that is apparent, not the architect. If the knowledge of Shapiro's relationship with Bernie Madoff were more concrete, if it were known definitively that Shapiro was in no way coerced, how would this further augment the $25 million already augmenting bodies inside the Shapiro Cardiovascular Center? Augmenting bodies both literally, surgically, and metaphorically, repositioning us. The obvious argument, given the beneficial ability to perform potentially life saving operations, is that it should just matter that the money is there, not where it came from. Even the billions at stake in the Madoff scheme is not blood money on the scale of war or conflict diamonds, for example. Perhaps "blood money" should include not only the blood shed in the gaining of the money but the blood saved by it. Or the blood created by it.

Smilow, Joel E. Smilow, that is, is also connected to blood, though in an admittedly tangential way. Playtex Sport, longest running competitor to Tampax, inventor of the plastic tampon applicator, is a key holding of Playtex Inc., the company Joel E. Smilow was the President and CEO of and where his money was made. A feminine blood money. Playtex also sells bras and many household products and counts among either its holding or business partners brands and companies ranging from Max Factor and Revlon to Procter & Gamble and Hanes. It is much too large a network to attempt to list everything here. It is as if Joel E. Smilow is more like an organization and less like an individual, personal, human.

There's nothing (seemingly) personal about Smilow Cancer Care Center either because, unlike Shapiro, there are no immediately apparent personal or familial relationships that seem slightly disarrayed. This is also, surely, a feeling influenced by the distinct impersonalness of the care at Smilow Cancer Care Center, an effect of its function as part of Yale New Haven Hospital, a teaching hospital.

Which means, pragmatically, that first you speak to one or more medical students who then speak, without you, to your doctor, who then all return to speak to you or to tell you what they discussed or to tell you what they have already decided before speaking to you. Maybe a classroom really wouldn't be better than a jury.

Emblem

Here is another way that I understand as a method (such as it is) of using my body to measure distance, one Emblem surely can't (or doesn't want) to understand: It is nearing the end of the year and it took me the past several weeks to bring myself to buy a new planner, one that extended past the next several months. It was not a question of money or opportunity. But if the distance between now and next week or now and when I am finally able to have the CT scan or now and whenever what the scan does or doesn't show is understood, cannot or may not be able to be contained by my body, how could the next year?

There it is again, a gothic-appropriate yearning. It is a feeling distinct to the gothic, to Lena's lust for pale female flesh. It's not a sentimentality, exactly, inasmuch as my awareness of it here is not one of embarrassment, like being embarrassed for seeming so melodramatic, but just a sense of fitting, almost ironic, yearning. So romantic, so gothic, and, yet, so bureaucratic. Which is, perhaps, exactly what the gothic refers to: desires of outsiders at a time of defining borders and morals and ideals, defining done by groups of people, government, media; bureaucracies.

It's not only about the outsiders though. The gothic is also about defining the groups themselves. And, specifically, the spaces these groups occupy; the gothic is the empty castle. "Who's Caring For You?" and the entire Emblem website is an empty castle. Consider again *Dracula* and the journey Dr. Van Helsing is able to take to come to Transylvania; the power of the empire as expressed through a mobile, border-crossing, physical presence. The power of Emblem as expressed through bright white margins, a URL; friendly, accessible, but something you must choose to enter into — Emblem is not coming to you. "Who's Caring For You?" attempts to counteract this very emptiness, the facelessness, the inability to define the monster that lies at the heart of the gothic narrative, by providing a face, many faces, people for you to get to know. But who do you really know besides Emblem Health HIP? And do you even really know them? When you call a customer service number and hear a recording tell you that you've reached Encore Health, formerly known as another health company whose name is also not Emblem, will you be surprised? How does an interaction with/in "Who's Caring For You?" compare to an interaction within a building named for a person? Both are sites that function as physical expressions of social, byzantine, networks and as host to the more personal, gothic, networks of those involved in the building itself. How does an attraction to the bright white space of "Who's Caring For You?" come to supplement the fluorescent lights in the Carl J. Shapiro Cardiovascular Center? Do I know Emblem Health or Carl J. Shapiro better? Who's caring for me?

I am not alone in my yearning. In regards to Emblem Health HIP I may be, but Carl J. Shapiro and Joel E. Smilow and Richard H. Nesson surely wanted something more than to be relieved of many millions of dollars. Nesson stands out in this regard, though, as the only one of the three for whom Brigham and Women's dedicated the building. He gave no money, but did serve as Hospital President for many years, overseeing the formation of a partnership with other area hospitals (Mass General, Boston Children's, Dana Farber; why do I know this from memory?) to form Partners Healthcare. A partnership that looks like a simultaneous huge expansion and solidification, a closing up of the castle. Because while it certainly succeeded in bringing healthcare to more people through community initiatives, Partners Healthcare also represents a consolidation of billions of dollars' worth of providers and the bodies they care for. And, to further solidify the importance of a few key hospitals, Partners Healthcare works with teaching and medical research centers run by Harvard University, thus ensuring that educational standards, once set, will be passed down. Classrooms and juries both.

Not that I mean to sound ungrateful. I am incredibly thankful to have access to the level of care I have/had at Brigham and Women's (disregarding current SNAFU) but just because Partners Healthcare or even Emblem Health HIP ultimately benefit many more people than not, doesn't mean that the ways in which their organizations are or become gothic networks should be disregarded, especially given the ways these networks affect physical bodies and are built into the spaces they move through. After all, so much has been done under the banner of the greater good that ultimately turned out to be not that good for anyone.

Fernald

Outside of the reoccurring castle motif it seems that, especially in more recent iterations of what are still gothic novels, the school is a common threatening or threatened space. One of the most gothic: The Walter E. Fernald School for Boys, in Waltham, Massachusetts. Still standing, but empty, the Fernald School is the oldest school in the country for boys with disabilities (or orphans). Waltham is not particularly far from where I live in Boston; its distance could be measured by the long walk it would take me to get there. Or, I could use my body to measure my distance to the Fernald School in a different way, because in the 1940s and 50s, the Fernald School was the site of ongoing experiments led by the Massachusetts Institute of Technology and Harvard University, for the United States government, funded by the Quaker Oats company. Experiments that were never acknowledged as such, experiments for which informed consent was never given by the parents of the boys involved, experiments that were run as the Boys' Science Club: a group of students who were treated with trips to baseball games and other outings and who were, additionally, given a breakfast every day that consisted of oatmeal that had been dosed with radiation.

I first learned about the Fernald School not because it's nearby but in a medical ethics textbook (as a case about informed consent in medical testing) as part of coursework. A few days after this, I went into the hospital (White Plains Hospital; no name that I remember) to have a gastric emptying scan, a procedure that begins when the radiology technician brings you a breakfast of an egg sandwich to which has been added radioactive material.

Ostensibly, the Fernald experiment was designed as a nutrition study, which I understand as an early attempt at what is now a commonplace item: fortified cereal. My understanding is a little lacking though because the information around the experiments is understandably lacking as well. When the Boys' Science Club was found out, in the 1990s, the surviving members pursued litigation that resulted in a $1.85 million settlement. It was difficult to prove in court how much of what kind of damage was done, with the United States government arguing that the amounts of radiation fed to the boys were no more than the amount of background radiation absorbed in a city during the course of a year.[6] Which is, I would imagine, a common difficulty and disadvantage in medical malpractice cases involving already sick people.

It was in a fairly common medical ethics textbook that I learned about the Fernald School. Maybe one used, today, by the Harvard School of Public Health or elsewhere within Partners Healthcare.

What kind of blood money was the settlement given to the Fernald School boys? More or less of the same kind of blood or money as the sponsorship originally provided by the Quaker Oats company? Blood money is not too strong a term because both the experiment itself and the lawsuit that followed are a form of violence. A "bureaucratic violence" which consists of "attacks on those who insist on alternative schemas or interpretations."[7] That is, like the borders of England against Dracula, the gothic bureaucracy must keep the in- and out-of-network state clear, precisely through such acts as governments, educational institutions and corporations deciding what bodies should or shouldn't be informed about the radiation they are or are not being administered.

Given the high stakes and violence involved in networks like those related to the Fernald School, what or whose purpose does it serve to rewrite a gothic romanticism into such relationships? My irradiated breakfast was a few years ago (and fully covered by Emblem Health HIP) but I do, now, remember that while eating an irradiated egg sandwich was not cool, exactly, it was certainly a novel experience. It was eerie. It was the first time that so many bureaucratic distances collapsed in(to) my body. Literally, into my body via not a distance but a number: a tracer dose, an amount of radiation, an amount given daily to the Fernald School boys and roughly equal to the doses given in nuclear medicine imaging studies today.

---

6 Zareena Hussain, "MIT to Pay Victims $1.85 Million in Fernald Radiation Settlement," *The Tech* 117.65, January 7, 1998, http://tech.mit.edu/V117/N65/bfernald.65n.html.

7 David Graeber, *The Utopia of Rules: On Technology, Stupidity, and the Secret Joys of Bureaucracy* (Brooklyn, NY: Melville House Press, 2015), 80.

Shapiro

It takes imagination to rewrite bureaucracies as gothic romances. This is important when the bureaucratic violence perpetrated in cases like the Fernald School boys is a product of a system in which bureaucracies are "ways of organizing stupidity—of managing relationships that are already characterized by extremely unequal structures of imagination."[8] Further, to follow the "Italian philosopher Giorgio Agamben [who] argued that from the perspective of sovereign power, something is alive because you can kill it,"[9] certain systems of bureaucratic violence are expressions of an inability to imagine that certain bodies are alive enough to be killed. It's telling that the experiments and subsequent revealing of them were under the auspices of the US Department of Energy, not the Department of Health and Human Services.

Is being in the Shapiro Cardiovascular Center or Smilow Cancer Care Center more like being in a building or being with a person? Is being in a gastric emptying scan more like being in an imaging suite or being with the bodies who helped (were used to) determine the safety of the scan for you? Is such a distinction really necessary or even possible, though? Who benefits from a separation of physical and social space except those for whom Carl J. Shapiro Cardiovascular Center should remain a life-saving building and not a building constructed by familial ties both nearly nepotistic and financially fraudulent? Who benefits from a separation of physical and social space if not those who fully understand that "deface" is something that can be done to both people and buildings?

Deface as in: spaces so faceless no amount of fluorescence or natural lighting can make them clear. Deface as in: on some imaging machines, like MRIs, one is in an internal space with small lights overhead but in nuclear imaging devices there are no lights and I remember the darkness of the ceiling lights, panels, of the room itself and I remember the darkness of the MIT newspaper website where I read about the Fernald School settlement and I remember that nowhere was bright enough for me to see the boys themselves. Deface as in: today, finally, the last of the necessary information

8   Graeber, *The Utopia of Rules,* 81.
9   Graeber, *The Utopia of Rules,* 86.

will be sent to Emblem Health HIP (in the continued aim of getting the CT scan, sometime) but whatever the blinking lights of the fax machine convey, my body remains out-of. Deface as in: Brigham and Women's has been under construction for all the years I've been going there; campuses and buildings have footprints as much as bodies do.

Deface as in: light is as much about creating reflections as it is about dispelling shadows. I was in a fluorescent-lit hallway at 6:45AM one month ago and the fluorescent lights were overhead but also in the shine of the floor and also in the heavy glass doors behind me and also now.

Coda

Yesterday I discovered that Emblem Health HIP has 45 one-star reviews on Yelp (to be clear: there are nothing *but* one-star reviews). I love them all. All seem to be complaints along such similar lines as mine: a doctor orders a test or a referral and Emblem declines to pay for it, and Emblem gives the complaint holder a runaround during any attempts to access customer service. Especially compared to the mostly inaccessible complaints on the Better Business Bureau website, these Yelp reviews are a kind of poetry. I love them all. These reviews are distinct from other Yelp pages, reviews of shops or businesses, because they are differently personal. Instead of the personal experience and indignation in a review concerning poor service in a store, for example, these reviews are tinged with outraged desperation; a long wait for dinner is one thing, a long way for a doctor's appointment entirely different. It is as if the Yelp reviewers of Emblem Health live in a world where it is permanently the summer, where health services are permanently staffed by first year medical students and the computer systems are always only changing. One reviewer writes that she read all of these one-star reviews and chose to sign up for (to buy) Emblem Health anyway, thinking that all insurance companies are bad. She writes that she was wrong, that she discovered a horror unique to Emblem Health. I love her especially. This love goes beyond vindication, because, anyway, is vindication even possible or fulfilled if Emblem Health continues to deny me? It is a love of humanness; the satisfaction of seeing the gothic facelessness of Emblem Health dissolve into a sea, a page, of very real people writing words very close to my own. It is a return of not only humanity, personality, to bureaucracy, but a return of imagination as well, a balancing of imagination. I can imagine exactly what it must have been like for the woman awaiting hip surgery or the person billed $1,800 for routine blood work ordered by an in-network doctor, and I know that they must, also, be able to imagine my own wait time, my own anonymous case numbers. All too well. Our own Emblem.

* * *

And, lastly, a final update a year after initially writing this essay, necessary now to fully consider the implications of my relationship to Emblem Health: I never received the CT scan my doctor originally ordered. Instead, an in-network doctor I had also been seeing recommended doing a colonoscopy, a procedure that would look at more or less the same area. I had none of what either of my doctors were looking for. What my doctor was not looking for, and which he had previously told me he would not find in a 22-year-old, but did find, was an adenoma—a small intestinal growth, like a mole, that develops into colon cancer if left in place. The CT scan my doctor originally wanted would not have found this growth; nothing would have been found, and no further tests would have similarly gone looking. Given that routine colonoscopies for colon cancer screening are not recommended until age 50, I feel it's safe to assume that I would never have had a colonoscopy and I would have had colon cancer by the time I was 30. "Who's Caring For You?"

Daily Survivor #1

Daily Survivor

The American Chronic Pain Association recommends making decoupage boxes (among other crafts) as a form of pain management.

Daily

If being in pain every day necessitates surviving said pain every day which (if successful) results in the state of being a daily survivor, how often or to what extant can "daily" build up on itself before completely obliterating any meaningful definition of "survivor"? What are the temporal dimensions of "survivor"?

Daily Survivor

The American Chronic Pain Association does not recommend doing manual labor for a living as part of a pain management strategy, especially for those who are legally disabled.

Survivor

Recently, much scholarly attention has been given to trauma, surviving trauma, and plasticity.[1] Plasticity meaning, very generally,

1   See Catherine Malabou, *Ontology of the Accident: An Essay on Destructive Plasticity* (Cambridge, UK: Polity, 2012) and Antonio Damasio, *Looking for Spinoza: Joy, Sorrow and the Feeling Brain* (San Diego, CA:

physical, mental, and specifically neurological changes and growth that occur in the aftermath of traumatic events (whether physical or mental to begin with). These new survivors, people left affectively different, either positively, neutrally, or negatively, are left as such after events that are exactly that: events, as in moments or accidents or temporal instances in some way limited by distinct parameters of time.

Daily

Does being a daily survivor imply that singular events happen every day which must be survived or that the very quality of daily-ness (which includes the qualities of ordinariness and unending repetition) is a traumatic event to be survived? Or, really, is it the pain that needs to be survived or the fact that it happens every day?

Daily Survivor

The American Chronic Pain Association does not recommend doing manual labor while legally disabled because that would be too much like fighting fire with fire (as opposed to decoupage boxes).

Daily

Although, actually, the hidden genius of decoupage boxes as a daily pain management strategy is that decoupage boxes are daily-ness itself and thus making decoupage boxes as a daily pain management strategy fully actualizes fighting fire with fire because both decoupage boxes and daily-ness itself are ubiquitous, all-accessible, everywhere, boring.

Daily Survivor

Being in pain every day is intensely boring.

Harcourt, 2003).

Daily

The trauma of daily-ness, as it is shaped by both ordinariness and temporal conditions of ceaselessness, is that it is boring. Being in pain daily, being in daily-ness, is boring because it is always the same (because the pain is always there) and also always changing (because the pain is never the same and because it is always a new day).

Daily Survivor

Being in pain every day is boring because it does not provide opportunities for personal growth and resiliency in the face of singular traumatic events.

Being in pain every day is boring as a problem deserving academic or scholarly attention because it does not provide opportunities for groundbreaking neurology and positive thinking and personal growth. Even as a problem examined within affect theory and by scholars who study ordinary life, being in pain every day isn't actually ordinary enough because it is only the realm of the already sick.

The American Chronic Pain Association does not admit that being in pain every day is boring nor do they give suggestions for managing this boredom. (Though decoupage boxes may be a form of admission.)

Survivor

The problem of the boringness of being in pain every day, and part of the reason this is a problem for scholars, is that there is no resiliency. Resiliency is inherently about sponginess, about bouncing back (to normal), about recovery. What kind of recovery is possible when what is wrong is wrong in the very daily-ness of one's existence?

Daily Survivor

In some ways, doing manual labor for a living as a pain management strategy follows the American Chronic Pain Association's boring logic, the logic of immersion in daily-ness as a way out of it, because manual labor is what the majority of people do on a daily basis.

As I write this, I am at the public library watching a landscaping crew mulch around trees outside. (Tomorrow I will load bags of mulch into people's cars as part of [one of] my jobs at a garden center.)

Daily

Being in pain every day is boring because boring is a quality that experiences have; boredom is the state of being bored. So saying "Being in pain every day is boring" is different from saying "I'm bored because I'm in pain every day" because the former identifies the pain as the thing which is boring, it does not mean that I'm bored.

Simultaneously, being is pain every day is boring means finding oneself unafraid, because you cannot be bored and afraid at the same time.

Daily Survivor

You can, however, find something boring and be angered by this boringness at the same time.

Daily

Would it be boring if it didn't happen every day? Would it be boring if it provided the groundwork for being able to make serious, resilient, personal growth? Would it be boring if I weren't so mad?

Daily Survivor

Being in pain every day is not about resiliency because when being in pain every day is the only daily state possible there is nothing to resiliently return to; when being in pain happens every day there is never, exactly, a daily return of the pain but simply a repetition. Being in pain every day instead becomes about stamina, because stamina is not about surviving moments or events but about surviving time itself.

Being bored by pain means not being afraid because you cannot be afraid (and waiting) to die and bored simultaneously. Being in pain and bored means not being afraid of dying (or being too bored to be afraid). But is being angry really any better?

Daily

This bored un-afraidness is not a death acceptance/relinquishing of existentialism because being bored is not about not caring or not taking the pain seriously or deciding to simply spend all your time making decoupage boxes. It is simply what happens when pain happens every day, when you know that pain as well as you know how to unthinkingly get up and make coffee and brush your teeth. The moment being in pain every day turns into being (in pain) every day, it's boring because do you really find getting up and making coffee and brushing your teeth to be that interesting?

Daily Survivor

Doing manual labor every day is also (sometimes) boring. But it is invaluable as a pain management strategy because if my legs and arms and feet are sore than my stomach hurts less (noticeably): and, I can remember how hard I worked the previous day when it is now the middle of the afternoon on a weekday and I am lying in bed with a hot water bottle and a book doing my other work.

Daily

Being in pain every day is a form of manual labor. This makes the application of words like "management" (i.e. "pain management") all the more applicable, because being in pain every day is a form of activity that you have to do and manage yourself in doing as you would any other job.

Especially when writing about being sick, writing based either overtly or subtly on being in pain every day, is your other work. Especially when you are contracted for this other work but not for the manual labor day jobs which fund your ability to be in pain and in bed the rest of the time.

Survivor

That being in pain every day is a form of manual labor downplays the significance or importance or value of your ability to survive because at this point you are just doing your job.

It does not, though, make being in pain every day any less boring. Because, ultimately, your task in this job is to simply get through it, to move through time.

Being in pain every day is a form of manual labor in which the hours are unpredictable but endless and ultimately the most precarious situation to find yourself in.

Daily Survivor

Being in pain every day is boring and boredom is not the worst feeling.

Survivor

In fact, boredom is preferable to many other feelings (namely fear) and can even be comforting. Because although being in pain every day with a certain consistency in that pain, there are still moments capable of causing fear or surprise or worry. Being bored is comforting when it means that the focus is on boredom and not on pain.

Being in pain every day, boringly, also means that the boredom itself can be painful, tedious. But even this kind of pain is still preferable.

Daily

Boring-ness is comforting because having everything (even pain) (especially pain) stay the same is preferable when change only means getting worse. Boring-ness is comforting when it means finding stability in a precarious situation.

Daily Survivor

Being in pain every day is boring because being in pain doesn't necessarily mean suffering; at least suffering would provide something to do.

Survivor

What does the manual labor of being in pain every day produce? The state of being a survivor. Which is intricately twined to the dual nature of the not interesting/tedious mental/physical nature of the boredom of being in pain every day, because it means that the manual labor of being in pain every day is a physical act which produces a mental state, the state of being a survivor.

Daily

Doing repetitive manual labor every day is not in and of itself precarious; Sisyphus could at least take a sick comfort in the fact that nothing about his situation was ever going to change (or get worse).

Daily Survivor

Being in pain every day is boring and it is an intense privilege to find oneself bored by this pain; this is part of the comfort of boredom, that when it is unending and repetitive it becomes a form of deep boredom. Deep boredom is not a transcendental form of boredom, because it doesn't make being in pain or being bored at all pleasurable. If anything, it is sub-boredom, so repetitive (and painful) that one cannot even build a narrative of having survived an individual episode of boredom. But deep boredom is still a privilege because being deeply bored and in pain still means not (being dead or) being in such pain as to be unable to be bored. I will take all the moments of boredom I can get.

Survivor

Part of the pain of boredom is some sense of shame at finding, ultimately, only boredom and no transcendence in being in pain every day. Being a survivor makes everyone, even and especially those who have nothing to survive (yet), feel better. Being bored helps no one. Which is, of course, the beauty and entertainment value of life-changing narratives; no one ever tells or is entertained by a narrative of life changed only by its very un-changing-ness.

Daily Survivor

Not only does it fully capture daily-ness, decoupage boxes are also an appropriate metaphor for the particular boredom of being in pain every day, because decoupage is about building up and affixing layers: if being in pain is like a blister, then being in pain every day and finding it boring is like a callus, because one is filled with something and the other only ever becomes more and more of itself, "it's Infinite contain."[2]

Daily

Layering up metaphors like decoupage boxes is the only kind of thinking possible about (and within) the boredom of being in pain every day: oblique. Because what is there when trying to face and think about boredom directly? Nothing (pain).

Survivor

Is the failure to craft or produce a narrative of survival a failure of the manual labor of being in pain every day or a failure of the mental (non)work of boredom?

Daily

Deep boredom is or can become a part of this oblique thinking, adding positively to it, because deep boredom is a form of attention. If boredom is characterized by an inability to find something capable of absorbing one's attention completely, deep boredom is a constant awareness of this inability to fully pay attention to a thing which itself is also always present.

---

2   Emily Dickinson, *The Complete Poems of Emily Dickinson* (Boston, MA: Little, Brown, 1924), 340.

Survivor

The manual labor of being in pain every day is precarious (in part) because it is not a job you are paid to do, but a job that you pay to do, with your attention.

Daily

Although deep boredom is about always partially paying attention to something (else, something you are not capable of giving your full attention to) it does not produce a state of being distracted. In fact, deep boredom prevents distraction because it constantly acknowledges present pain and how boring it would be to fully be in this pain and what a distraction this pain would become.

Daily Survivor

Deep boredom in which pain is paid attention to and always already displaced (by boredom, by not fully paying attention, by refusing to be distracted) is a way of being a daily survivor.

Survivor

On the other hand, deep boredom and an ability to not fully find oneself immersed in the manual labor of being in pain every day means always constantly having to find other things to pay attention to, anything better than being in pain (even boredom).

Death is a Deadline

Being in pain every day, because it is boring, because this boredom must be managed, is a problem not only of pain management but of time management as well. Because, after all, "Death is like a deadline."[3]

---

3   "For Man with Cystic Fibrosis, 'death is like a deadline'," *National Public Radio,* May 1, 2015, http://www.npr.org/2015/05/01/403303311/for-man-with-cystic-fibrosis-death-is-like-a-deadline.

Daily

Having a deadline implies having a product that must be due by that time. The deadline of death means optimizing your pain and time management strategies to produce a narrative of how well you survived before you die.

Death is a failure of management.

Survivor

This deadline shouldn't be a problem, though, because being bored, especially being in deep boredom, doesn't mean doing nothing. Except that optimized management and being a survivor in the face of the deadline of death isn't enough: optimized management, especially of time, should result not only in narrative production but in the production of productivity itself.

Death is a Deadline

But what kind of time management is possible when being in pain every day is boring and does not come with a set or definite disease-related life expectancy? Or, what is the difference between life expectancy as an amount of time and life expectancy as a quality of time?

Daily Survivor

Or, as my coworker put it when telling me about how, upon learning of her rheumatoid arthritis diagnosis, all but one of her professors recommended finding an alternate career to horticulture and landscaping: sometimes in chronic illness it is not just chronic illness but also chronic bullshit.

Death is a Deadline

The chronic bullshit of being in pain every day and finding it boring is a kind of life expectancy.

Survivor

How does anticipating having to survive a quality instead of an amount of time change what it means to be a daily survivor?

Daily

The problem of the boredom of being in pain every day stems not just from the pain itself but from how boring (almost) everything else, like decoupage boxes, seems in the face of said pain. This boredom is inseparable from the anger it produces. Why isn't anything interesting enough? Why suggest decoupage boxes as an alternative, as if it were really that easy?

Death is a Deadline

Here is an example of the quality that is my life expectancy and the way that I will find it taxing, as in, the way I will have to pay, which is with my attention. Like when I find myself non-bored, reading Donald Hall's *Life Work* until I am derailed by the sentence "And then Jack found a problem in his abdomen" and I will not remember or pay attention to anything past that on page 8.[4]

Daily Survivor

Although being dead is presumably even more boring.

When "life itself has been put to work," when the pain and boredom of being in pain every day becomes a form of manual labor to which the rules of pain and time management can (must) be applied, what sort of work ethic is possible?[5] Just as the problem of being in pain every day is not just about pain but about boredom, the question of a work ethic is about both how to do this kind of manual labor but also about how to ethically hold a position that is predicated on the privilege of being able to find pain boring.

---

4   Donald Hall, *Life Work* (Boston, MA: Beacon Press, 1993), 8.
5   Michael Hardt and Antonio Negri, *Declaration* (New York: Argo-Navis Author Services, 2012), 12.

Daily

Time management includes not just time but the larger area of logistics management, how to move stuff and schedule this moving: how to schedule procedure appointments so they interfere with neither your vacation time nor your (day job) work schedule.

Daily Survivor

Having a strong work ethic is an intrinsic part of the American dream because it's the route to all success. Despite having however many day jobs and other work, being in pain every day and sick is my all-the-time job. Manual labor, definitely, but this job also involves affective and caring labor. A kind of affective labor closely aligned with (historically) feminine, mothering (invisible) forms of labor, oft taken for granted and long discounted as being actual work. The problem in applying the term "logistics" here, therefore, is that the scale is wrong, because logistics is inherently about massive quantities; it is this mass which institutes the necessity of management. The work of being in pain every day is intensely, specifically, domestic.

Daily

Before moving on, though, to questions of a work ethic and care labor and the work of being in pain every day, I feel the need to further clarify this notion of boredom, though that itself may seem redundant and boring. But it's because I'm not quite getting it. Yes, being in pain every day is boring and this boredom involves anger and work and time management and attention and it becomes such an embedded part of daily life that it seems not just like a job but like deep boredom: an unending almost non-boring daily-ness that takes work to maintain. But it's exactly this work that I've neglected. Because there is, on the one hand, the very manual labor of being in pain and the affective work necessary to do this pain/work more easily around others, and then, less manually, less physically, there is the work of boredom, the mental and affective work needed to negotiate the constant daily resource drain (on attention, energy) that being in pain every day becomes. This work of boredom is pure, banal, management, a kind of anti-mindfulness wherein part of the process is always about ignoring something, ignoring physical pain or anger or those decoupage boxes that seem like the only alternative. Or, perhaps, it's a death deadline-specific kind of mindfulness. Or, it is nothing more than logistics management at its most domestic level, because it is entirely a working life spent "simplifying or accelerating functions of unreasonable banality."[6]

Life's Work

Life's working means (having to) work to make life.

Daily Survivor

Being a daily survivor is work. In addition to all the aforementioned qualities and conditions of this work, it is, absolutely, a work of narrative. It is work in the form of saying "being a daily survivor is work." It is work in the form of saying "I am an invalid."

Life's Work

Finding one's life work, coupled with or driven by or dependent on one's work ethic, is also a key part of the American dream process. Even when one doesn't or is unable to choose one's life work and is instead, simply, (simply?) made to have one?

Daily Survivor

Being a daily survivor is a form of life's work because it is sometimes the only way to make life (work).

Survivor

But, on the other hand, a very big part of the anger inherent in the boredom of being in pain every day is anger at the commoditization

---

6   Alain De Botton, *The Pleasures and Sorrows of Work* (New York: Pantheon Books, 2009), 44.

of this kind of pain and the way that commoditization results in the products of heroic survivor narratives.

I am not that kind of daily survivor.

Life's Work

In a way, having one's life work chosen for you is an easier starting point than having to start from nothing because it means not feeling pressured to seek redemption or transcendence through work, when, as Donald Hall says, "Work is not redemptive...but it is or can be devoted."[7]

Daily Survivor

What is the object of devotion required for the work of being a daily survivor? Is being devoted affected, as in, is the quality or outcome of that devotion affected by whether or not it's actual devotion or an obligation? Is boredom always already apathy?

Life's Work

The work of writing "being a daily survivor is work" is sometimes work that I do while on my legally mandated half-hour break at my other manual labor day job.

Survivor

By refusing to work towards a heroic survivor narrative, am I a slacker?

Daily Survivor

The labor of being in pain every day is hard work but, simultaneously, hard work is the answer to being in pain every day.

7   Hall, *Life Work,* 9.

Pain Exists for a Reason

The reason being that pain "provides us with a built-in warning." The pain and boredom of being in pain every day is a warning against that very boredom.

Daily

Actually, not the exact same boredom of being in pain every day. It is instead a warning of the boredom and pain of not being in (this) pain, of the absence of (the necessity of) hard work. As counterintuitive as this may seem, "pain free" doesn't always really mean free. Because if you have worked to make your life('s work), what is the cost of losing that?

Pain Exists for a Reason

On the other hand, chronic pain as experienced by millions of Americans costs "$635 billion a year in medical care and lost labor."[8]

Daily

While the pain of being in pain every day does carry its own warning, if your pain is caused by or a part of a chronic illness, there's no real risk in that chronic ceasing.

Daily Survivor

Is the term "lost labor" meant to indicate a withdrawal from the workforce by people who are in pain or does "lost" also carry implications of the fact that care labor, the labor of being in pain every day, is always already lost both because it is not generally considered valuable and because lost can imply invisible or otherwise out of sight?

---

8   Stephani Sutherland, "Pain That Won't Quit," *Scientific American,* December 2014, 62, http://www.erythromelalgia.org/Portals/0/ProspectsforTreatingChronicPainScientificAmerican.pdf.

Daily

My other manual non-lost labor is worth approximately $12/hour (before taxes). My other manual non-lost labor provides more of an income than disability benefits would.

Pain Exists for a Reason

Pain exists as a way of providing work to people who (may) need it.

Survivor

In a review of the television show *The Unbreakable Kimmy Schmidt,* the critic Emily Nussbaum identifies the protagonist as practicing a "powerfully girlish model of toughness."[9]

Pain Exists for a Reason

Pain exists a way to provide a powerfully disabled model of toughness.

Daily

The muscles I develop at my manual labor day job are not exactly strong enough to mend internal organs.

Pain Exists for a Reason

Maybe, actually, pain really just reinforces a "girlish model of toughness" because chronic pain is more prevalent among women than men and because (in part) (talking about) being in pain is more often associated with being a wimp than a laborer and wimps are girlish.

---

9   Emily Nussbaum, "Candy Girl," *The New Yorker,* March 30, 2015, http://www.newyorker.com/magazine/2015/03/30/candy-girl.

Daily

Maybe pain and its lost labor only reinforces girlishness because lost labor is already in the realm of the feminine in that invisible care labor is predominantly done by women.

Pain Exists for a Reason

The kind of pain that provides a girlishness-reinforcing disabled model of toughness is not daily pain nor the pain of dailyness but is only ever other people's pain. Specifically, other people's pain as expressed in heroic survivor narratives.

Survivor

By refusing to work towards a heroic survivor narrative am I a slacker? Or, am I a slacker simply because the work that I do in being in pain every day is unseen?

Daily Survivor

Not entirely unseen by everyone, though, because there is that coworker, and other coworkers as well, other women employed in multiple forms of chronic labor.

Life's Work

Other coworkers of a kind, because I am thinking of people I do not necessarily work with, but who I know to also be engaged in the work of being in pain every day. The thing about having coworkers in this work, though, is that as much solidarity as can be felt, there is also always a sense that when working to make one's life('s work), it is impossible to fully escape the particularities of that life and the work that must be done.

Daily Survivor

When I say that hard work is the answer to the (other) work of being in pain every day, I do not mean the kind of moralizing goodness of working hard, the kind of moral superiority of self-made men, but that hard work is as good an alternative as decoupage boxes.

Daily

Except in times like these when I am sitting in the library (on my day off) and it is (becoming) very clear that lost labor really only means exactly that — because I am in pain and distracted and anticipating more pain and there is no work that I will be able to get done, hard or otherwise.

Daily Survivor

Hard work is as good an alternative to decoupage boxes as any because it means that my coworkers and I are firmly in the opposite camp as bed-ridden invalid non-workers. Hard work is as good an alternative as decoupage boxes because valuing my labor as it is expressed in a decorative craft project meant only for my consumption means valuing my body as something capable of only that kind of pseudo-production.

Pain Exists for a Reason because Death is a Deadline for Life's Work

Maybe decoupage boxes would actually be harder than working hard because decoupage boxes seem to imply having to find value inherent in pain instead of value in the things pain allows you to do.

Dead-End Job

Maybe. Or maybe only a slacker in a dead-end job. That is, a slacker made such by the very predetermined unnecessariness of the job. Unnecessary not because the work itself is unneeded but because the dead-endedness of it renders any given task or larger project (slightly) null and void; even a survivor narrative is only valid until rendered invalid by the way that being dead means not surviving.

Daily

The other aspect of being, feeling like, a slacker in this job is the way that being in pain every day becomes automatic. Not the automation of robots capable of taking over your job, but the way that certain physical functions, like pain, automate you. In multiple ways. In the logistical sense of requiring the same basic care functions daily. But also the kind of automation implied by states and attitudes towards states like, for example, PMS, wherein menstruation explains away any "craziness." (Certain) biological functions absolve you of the responsibility for certain emotional states; it's only PMS.

It's only the pain talking.

Daily Survivor

Being in pain every day is a boring dead-end job that absolves you of having to be apologetic about the anger, frustration, boredom or general old cranky reclusive-ness that may result.

Daily

Having a dead-end job doesn't mean having no work, though, because it is still something you're employed in doing, and thus can be considered a "filled present," wherein "activity and speed distinguish the filled present, rather than emotional investment."[10] Simultaneously, the speed that characterizes a filled present may actually be a lack thereof.

Survivor

In the same way that biological functions explain away emotional states, they also invalidate emotions that may, actually, not be inherent. Thinking that it's only the pain talking renders the pain-having person mute. This is the truth of the process of automation within a dead-end job: having a dead-end job means your agency has become dead-ended, means you are now just a body that does a thing (to

10 Kathy Charmaz, *Good Days Bad Days* (New Brunswick, NJ: Rutgers University Press, 1993), 241.

you), that is in pain every day, that bores you and creates mounting bored-frustration which threatens your ability to project (affect) manage.

What, exactly, is the thing that has to be survived about being in pain every day? Is the pain or the boredom worse? Is the fact that thinking about, writing about, being in pain every day necessitates, always, the use of analogy and the laying of other systems over this pain, a symptom of the boredom or an inability to deal directly with certain physical experiences? When trying to think about what it is to survive is an ongoing thing, how can this thinking ever not reset at the end of any day? As in, how can the idea of being a survivor lengthen or expand to encompass a span of time longer than 24 hours? This is why "survivor" seems, as a concept, suited only to people who go through and come fully out of a singular event. Because when you are going through and coming (maybe fully, probably only partially) out of only a day at a time, how is this at all different from just being alive?

Daily Survivor

It's different because of the pain. It's different because while "being a survivor" is better suited to singular events, "surviving" can imply an ongoing process, without end, with an ongoing set of emotional processes tied to singular survived events as well as to the affective work of the everyday. This everyday is never, can never, be ordinary (as in normal) but is also simultaneously intensely ordinary, because it happens every day and because pain is, actually, intensely ordinary because it is only ever what (all) bodies do.

Given these parameters of survivorship, what is the measure of success in this job of being in pain every day? Some hugely meaningful end product or simply the drive to create, to work hard at, one? But this all too often is the only mark of successful survivorship, the mark of emotional strength and a best-selling memoir and a foundation in your name. None of this is meaning. Which is why, in addition to actually dying at the end, being in pain every day is a dead-end job: the oppression inherent in the way that certain kinds of survivors are lauded, renders anything you do, as not that kind of survivor, slightly pointless. Or not pointless, exactly, but meaningless in the eyes of a society that has chosen to value images (of success) over being alive (and knowing when that is success enough).

Survivor

But, at the end of the (this) day, who really can judge you when your only real coworker in the job of being in pain every day is your pain itself?

Wellness as Metaphor

Many times I have seen written the phrase "illness as metaphor." I have mostly seen it written like this: *Illness as Metaphor, Illness as Metaphor, Illness as Metaphor.* Because it is, or was, the name of a book, but now, through being written so many times, it is just illness as metaphor.

But illness is a thing that really happens. And aren't metaphors supposed to be narratives about the only way an unimaginable thing has become possible? Or maybe that's myth: "finding a hidden plot in a metaphor."[1]

Since illness is a thing that really happens, how can it be said that illness as metaphor is still the whole myth or still the only narrative through which to imagine a possible unimaginability? Since illness is a thing that really happens, where is the metaphor of opposing belief, the myth that illness never happens as a metaphor or as a real thing? A different or opposite or non-metaphor of illness isn't the same as a narrative about how illness never happens. To be a perfect myth about the absence of illness, illness can never be mentioned, as a myth or a metaphor or anything else. It must be something else.

It must be wellness.

Wellness feels good. Wellness feels like smoothies and coconut and January all year and whole foods and natural foods and local foods and organic foods. Wellness feels clean. Wellness feels like clean living, like a detox or like a tonic or like an elimination diet or like getting toxins out of your system. Wellness feels anti-inflammatory. Wellness feels so anti-inflammatory it is "cancer-free;" "getting to

1   Charles Simic, *The Monster Loves His Labyrinth: Notebooks* (New York: Ausable Press, 2008), 47.

the root of all disease;" "anti-aging." Wellness is good for you. But wellness is delicious and indulgent and decadent and never *tastes* good for you. Wellness is a practice of living. Wellness is homemade. Wellness is for life.

But: what, exactly, are toxins? This is never clearly defined: I have yet to see in any wellness-related media a list of bacteria or pathogens that accumulate in your body, cause demonstrable harm, and can be removed through things like "tonics." Especially as tonics can consist of anything from lemon and cayenne pepper in water to raw apple cider vinegar. Or they may even be a juice cleanse, which, again, can be anything from a drink that is more or less fiber to one that is more or less entirely sugar. Whether through a tonic or a juice cleanse, toxins are subject to being flushed out of the body. This is, in fact, already the job of several organs, notably the kidneys, liver, and intestines: human excrement can contain as many as 8 million bacterial cells. This is a design feature of the human body, one utilized with little to no additional support necessary from lemon water. In other cases, "toxins" can also include more deeply embedded or imperceptible substances, like the toxins that are found in or leach into your body through plastic, iPhones, cans, food packaging of any kind, multiple kinds of cookware, water, proximity to industrial or urban sources of pollution, pesticides, fruit or vegetables grown in non-organic conditions, as well as several other sources (all of which cause cancer).

The well body is at a surprising amount of risk for being so healthy.

Wellness, when it feels like January all year, full of commitment and resolutions, as well as during everyday practices of clean living and shorter periods like a detox, is an amount of time. As an amount of time which is assigned as a period during which certain tasks should be accomplished (i.e. "3-day juice cleanse"), wellness is work. But wellness is doing what you love: when periods of time are assigned for the completion of tasks that include the preparation of decadent and indulgent foods that are toxin-free, clean versions of common baked goods (by virtue of being wheat-, dairy-, soy- or egg-free), or the creation of decorative objects made by hand, such as wildflower arrangements or plant hangers (thereby reaping the benefit of increased exposure to oxygen-producing, air-toxin-cleaning plants as well as avoiding toxins in mass produced goods), then wellness never feels like work. This is further enhanced by the fact that wellness is, above all, a form of consumption. Not only because clean living necessitates the purchase of specialty clean ingredients or products, but also because it necessitates the consumption of wellness-focused media. Wellness requires instruction. As a set of practices that encompasses food, exercise, time management and consumption, wellness is labor as leisure. Wellness is unpaid labor that one does, actually, pay for, but it's always a fair price: wellness is its own reward.

Wellness is also many objects in and of themselves, mostly as conveyed through images and inspirational merchandising: mason jars, fresh fruit and vegetables in whole pieces or cut decoratively, especially as arranged by color or in an ombre pattern; natural fibers, particularly linen and wool, in muted earth or jewel tone colors; beeswax; bees themselves; wooden spoons; ceramics; hand-made ceramics; handmade ceramics in slightly unusable forms but nonetheless filled with decadent clean foods; Edison bulbs; any type of plant; candles; branches; coconuts; gym clothes that do not look like gym clothes; denim; flower arrangements; flower arrange-ments in mason jars; flower arrangements in repurposed Edison bulbs; bright light and aerial, overhead, shots (so as to better illus-trate the body's/viewer's position over the objects and therefore the body being in an optimal position to consume); also the Whole Foods bag (paper) printed with "Healthy Looks Good on You;" also the Whole Foods bag (reusable) printed with "Kale Quinoa Chocolate."

Wellness is a consumer good, and, like other forms of consump-tion, it is or has become a responsibility. Wellness is just the right thing to do.

Wellness is also much more than this. These are just the objects, images, and vocabulary through which it is communicated. Through these objects, images, and vocabulary wellness has become, if not by this exact name itself, still instantly recognizable as a lifestyle and perspective or rhetoric. Wellness means much more than its objects; it is, of course, a metaphor.

But continuing to examine the social practices through which it is expressed can yield valuable insights. As Susan Sontag writes in *Illness as Metaphor*: "Responses to illnesses associated with sinners and the poor invariably recommended the adoption of middle-class values."[2] Money drives the practices of wellness and makes its objects available. And to update Sontag's observation, written in the 1970s, it is only appropriate that now, in a time of a dissolving middle class, the practices and objects of wellness are not just moderately more expensive than cheaper versions of comparable goods: they are hugely inflated. But wellness as class marker is not purely economic, as Sontag continues: "With a slow motion epidemic, these same precautions take on a life of their own. They become part of social mores, not a practice adopted for a brief period of emergency, then discarded."[3] Wellness is for life.

When *Illness as Metaphor* was getting written over and over again and dissolving into illness as metaphor, into a taken-for-granted condition of an unimaginable thing or a thing that never happens — or a thing that only happens "in theory" or in literature — where was wellness? I imagine wellness circling around illness (as metaphor), looking for a way in, through the mass of cancer as uncontrolled growth metaphors or the invisible but difficult to pierce layer of AIDS as alien invasion. But these diseases are not part of the objects, focus, or concern of wellness. Wellness is not a metaphor or a narrative about the kinds of things cancer or AIDS were used to discuss, which changed over time but mainly consisted of fears about industrialization, capitalism, immigration, homosexuality and shifting cultural values. Wellness is not a narrative about any diseases, really; it is protection against them. Wellness is for life. This does not mean that there are not diseases lurking around the edges of wellness (perhaps just as wellness circled illness). These diseases on the fringes of wellness are those (thought to be) caused primarily by exposure to toxins and immersion in unclean environments, namely: autism and autoimmune diseases.

The relationship among autism, autoimmune diseases, and wellness centers around the idea of exposure to toxins. Blatantly, that exposure to toxic substances causes the body to malfunction on a deep, almost mysterious level. Both autism and many autoimmune diseases remain poorly explained in terms of pathophysiology, specifically in terms of triggers and causes. There are numerous models

2   Susan Sontag, *Illness as Metaphor and AIDS and its Metaphors* (New York: Farrar, Strauss and Giroux, 1978), 142.
3   Sontag, *Illness as Metaphor,* 162.

of "the autistic brain," none of which have been conclusively proven, especially given the wide variety or scale of autistic individuals. Likewise, autoimmune diseases and specifically those that develop later in life and frequently present as or include various kinds of food allergies or intolerances (or other environmental allergies), which are most often the focus within a wellness model of autoimmune diseases, also remain poorly explained. Most often the reason given within the personal narratives found on wellness-focused blogs and within popular science or health journalism is that contemporary crops are toxic, whether because of GMOs or pesticides or simply the fact that "modern humans" are not "designed" to eat certain foods. The high incidence of food allergy and autoimmune narratives in wellness is self-perpetuating: autoimmune diseases take years, on average, to diagnose, during which time people may be more likely to reach a stage of holistic, "natural" remedies than they would be if given more prompt, accessible and clearly explained medical treatment. Being more likely to participate in this kind of media makes the incidence of food allergies or autoimmune diseases seem disproportionately high; it also makes it seem like practices that people with documented medical problems need to do are things that all people should do, regardless of how well they may be to begin with. The standards for wellness are thus an inspirational goal for every body while paradoxically being set by those who are the least well.

On the other hand, within a wellness rhetoric, autism is easily explained: autism is caused by vaccines. Despite study after study and the personal statements of scientists involved in the initial research that clearly document the deep and unethical flaws incurred, a 1998 study showing correlation between the MMR (mumps, measles, and rubella) vaccine and autism continues to be taken as fact. This is not actually very different from a few of the narratives of illness that Susan Sontag cites in *Illness as Metaphor*: Turgenev's *On The Eve,* where "the hero of the novel realizes he can't return to Bulgaria...he sickens with longing and frustration, gets TB, and dies"; *Uncle Tom's Cabin,* wherein Little Eva is able to "announc[e] to her father a few weeks before the end," and then promptly die at the announced time; or James Joyce's *The Dead,* when "he said he did not want to live and a week later he dies."[4] Wellness, too, is an easy explanation.

It is not really accurate to say that wellness only makes it seem like food intolerances and autoimmune diseases are hugely common because they are, in fact, increasing in incidence rates. And it is also true that there has yet to be a proven explanation for this rise in related diseases. But it is still not inaccurate to say that wellness attracts people who have or think they have one of these conditions and, furthermore, that the rise in autoimmune diseases makes it that much more likely for a person consuming wellness media to know someone with an autoimmune disease or allergy. Autoimmune diseases and allergies are very real. At the same time, not only because they remain poorly understood but also because the array of symptoms such conditions can cause is vast, it makes it seem that much more likely that only something foreign to the body, something unidentifiably toxic, could cause this much damage. This is further reinforced by the frequent invisibility of both cause and the condition itself. As Sontag writes: "The marks on the face of the leper, the syphilitic, someone with AIDS, are signs of a progressive mutation, decomposition; something organic."[5] An absence of visible signs makes it all the easier for it to seem like something inorganic is happening.

Wellness is good and feeling good and looking good but it also allows for or asks for necessarily strong, almost harsh, discipline. This is obvious in the kinds of measures suggested for failure in everyday practices (i.e. the 30-day cleanse post-holiday season) as well as in responses to the perceived toxic inorganicness of autoimmune diseases and food intolerances. One need look no further than "gluten-free" to see a prime example of this attitude. "Gluten-free" is a set of dietary practices that involves a complete removal of gluten, a protein found in wheat and other grains, from one's diet, in addition to the purchase of specialty "gluten-free" or "certified gluten-free" items and the preparation, at home, of "gluten-free" recipes utilizing said "gluten-free" ingredients in order to create a perfect simulation of foods that do, in fact, contain gluten. In other words, the best and most well way to be "gluten-free" is to do it by

4   Sontag, *Illness as Metaphor*, 22–24.
5   Sontag, *Illness as Metaphor*, 129.

buying and spending time preparing things that make it seem like there is no absence of gluten whatsoever. Like you are giving up nothing. Like "gluten-free" is identical to living with gluten, only more well.

It would be easy to dismiss "gluten-free" as just another fad diet if not for three key features. First, because "gluten-free" is a set of practices involving consumption, labor, and social activity, all of which is, crucially, tied to a set of beliefs, it encompasses far more than other fad diets. The set of beliefs involved centers on a conviction about the toxicity of GMOs or the toxicity of modern wheat or the toxicity of modern agriculture and food processing. Because it is not just a diet, "gluten-free" is also not just or at all about weight loss. It is about feeling better. This feature also highlights the way in which sub-practices of wellness can and do dovetail with other forms of lifestyle-beliefs; in this case, the emphasis on feeling well and de-emphasis on weight loss, even through diet, align closely with mindful eating practices and the "Health at any size" movement. Lastly, "gluten-free" differs from fad diets like low-fat or low-carb because those diets encompass, essentially, all foods and by their very names suggest limited but still present quantities of the vilified substance. "Gluten-free," on the other hand, demands complete eradication of a single protein found in a handful of grains. There is no scale or level of acceptability: only total eradication. "Free."

Total eradication in the face of mysterious, inorganic, toxin-caused disease is the mechanism at the heart of most wellness practices. Wellness urges not only "gluten-free" but also: many other forms of eradication diets (Whole30, paleo, refined-sugar free), technology-free time periods, clutter-free living (see: Marie Kondo and the cult therein),[6] reducing plastic items entering the home, and so on. All of the practices and the media surrounding them are self-perpetuating and assert, over and over, that clean living is all that's needed. Wellness thereby denies the reality of illness and asserts itself as the only condition: if you live well (if you really live well and clean and do the detoxes and cleanses in the event of mistakes), then you will not get (these) illnesses. The wellness body is the prevented body.

6   See Marie Kondo's website: http://tidyingup.com/.

Prevention is a privilege. It is somewhat remarkable that, within wellness media, chronic illness seems a privilege as well. On the one hand, it is true that by the middle of the 20th century, "adults who would have previously died of infectious diseases were saved by sulphanomides and postwar antibiotics and thus moved on to the diseases of middle and old age."[7] Living long enough to get the kinds of disease frequently characterized as chronic is indeed a privilege. On the other hand, this flies in the face of epidemiological morbidity research that clearly demonstrates the correlation between illnesses like obesity, for example, and conditions of systemic oppression like poverty: chronic illness, of some kinds, very much does not come from living in and with privilege. How, then, does wellness figure chronic illness as a privilege? It is an impression gathered based on the various kinds of illness mentioned most frequently within wellness: food intolerances are the perfect example here. Not just because this is a chronic condition that generally requires little to no medical treatment perhaps beyond consultation: a food intolerance is a condition that can be managed entirely through diet and lifestyle. Like through buying specialty "certified gluten-free" items and having the leisure time to do so. Also, inasmuch as a food intolerance is distinct from a food allergy, a condition characterized by an immune system response that can result in emergency states like anaphylactic shock, a food intolerance is not deadly. And what a privilege being sick in this way is (provided there is no actual economic hardship preventing the purchase of "certified gluten-free" or other needed products, a hardship never mentioned in wellness). Additionally, chronic illness in wellness is a privilege because of the kinds of disease *not* mentioned therein: heart disease, obesity, stroke, hereditary diseases, diseases of old age, degenerative conditions, other physical disabilities. Not mentioned: diseases associated with poor people, people of color or other marginalized populations, that could have been prevented if given enough education (obesity, heart disease) or could never have been fully prevented in the first place (genetic diseases, short of genetic diseases caused by genes being turned on because of toxic exposures). It is as if wellness can only imagine and discuss diseases it would be a privilege to

7   George Weisz, *Chronic Disease in the 20th Century: A History* (Baltimore, MD: Johns Hopkins University Press, 2014), 8.

have when compared to many other, unimaginable, diseases. The well body is only "likely" to get certain diseases related to exposure to toxins and never anything associated with less privileged populations — many of whom may indeed be exposed to toxins as a result of economic, geographic, and racial discrimination, as in the recent case of lead contamination in the water of Flint, MI. "Considering illness as a punishment is the oldest idea of what causes illness."[8]

Discussing privilege within wellness necessitates a larger discussion of the well body. Thus far, the objects, practices, and images associated with wellness have been identified, but who purchases them, participates in, and aspires to these things? What are the characteristics of the well body? And it is a clearly definable body, especially when extrapolating from these images and related content, just as there was often a clearly identifiable body that was illness (as metaphor). For example, tuberculosis produced a body in which "debility was transformed into languor," with illness becoming "a kind of interior décor of the body," analogous to clothing.[9] In short, tuberculosis was inseparable from the aristocratic, artistic, and highly romanticized individual it produced. This individuality was so valued and idealized during the Romantic period that Sontag details, and this idealization fueled the production of a tuberculosis body during a time period in which rapid industrialization and a dissolving aristocracy meant that class markers like these could be entirely constituted visually. Furthermore, it was not only the bodies of those who actually had tuberculosis that were marked by it. The delicacy, paleness and thinness of the TB body continued to influence fashion well into the 20th century — see: heroin chic.

The well body's defining characteristics are its hypersensitivity and vulnerability to the environment. This contrasts with the simultaneous trait of physical fitness, usually expressed by participation in yoga, Soul Cycle, or related activities (Soul Cycle, in fact, seems to have such strong support within wellness it could easily be said that Soul Cycle is the new sanatorium). The hypersensitive nature combines with fitness to reinforce the requirement that the well body surround itself with clean organic objects, as much to avoid exposure as to support its level of fitness. Through this

8 Sontag, *Illness as Metaphor,* 133.
9 Sontag, *Illness as Metaphor,* 29.

hypersensitivity and fitness, the well body is thin and pale, but more so, it is the epitome of health: wellness is the glowing body.

Through this aesthetic, wellness marks a body with a very particular blend of vulnerability and fitness, presenting a hypersensitive feminine whiteness. These are class markers that further mark a body as one with ample leisure time and income (for paying for and attending yoga, Soul Cycle, specialty grocery stores, farmers markets, time for participating in wellness media itself): this leisure time and income is in no way wasted on the well body. It recognizes its purchasing power and votes with its dollars (see: the rapid shift among large food companies to incorporate cage-free eggs, natural, non-GMO, or fair trade items into their product lines) and has the education to do so. In short, the well body is one that can continually attend to and get the very best for its own support and care (out of choice and leisure and not out of medical necessity or debilitating illness). Wellness is its own pursuit.

Wellness is a body glowing with good health, but it is crucial here to draw a distinction between health or healthy and wellness. Doing so is best supported by providing an example of a prototypical well body: Carol, the protagonist in Todd Hayne's 1995 film *Safe,* played by Julianne Moore. Living in Los Angeles, Carol suddenly finds herself suffering from bizarre attacks: headaches, nose bleeds, shortness of breath. These attacks come seemingly at random, when a new couch is delivered to her house or as she is driving or at a baby shower. One day, Carol sees a flyer for a talk being given about something called environmental illness, and having received little to no treatment from both her doctor and psychiatrist, she decides to attend. The talk she hears not only confirms Carol's illness (as environmental) but provides much needed support, emotional support she had not been receiving from her husband or doctors, who seem mostly to consider her illness hysterical and psychosomatic. But it's not. And it is worth noting that it is only around this time, as Carol becomes sicker, but more importantly as she learns more about environmental illness, that bruises begin appearing on her face. As if, like the marks on a leper, now that the disease is known, definite and organic, what had been invisible can be made manifest and clearly marked, and can seem organic.

It may seem paradoxical to suggest that Carol, a sick person, is the prototypical well body. But she is exactly this body, like a resuscitated poster child. Carol asserts the importance and valid-ity of wellness through her very physicality, by demonstrating that (even in the absence of a single identifiable cause or source) "environmental" toxins can and will make you ill. Carol asserts the supremacy of wellness as a rhetoric as well, inasmuch as her turn away from her family and traditional medicine and towards the environmentally ill group she finds, ultimately going so far as to move to a retreat center the group runs, demonstrates that those around you may never believe in and validate a hypersensitive vul-nerable nature: only wellness is really there for you. Carol goes beyond just the wealthy, white, sensitive femininity that represents wellness so well, because her experience of finding a community run by people who have had the same experiences she has demonstrates a core wellness value: the need for communities led by individuals who have been through it themselves, and the value of the indi-vidual experience turned expert advice. This expert advice and the fact that wellness requires instruction is exactly what distinguishes wellness from healthy. Healthy is the FDA, myplate.gov, salad bars, a gym; healthy is mediocre. Healthy is mediocre because of its insis-tence on democracy and accessibility, especially when compared to the exclusive, individualized, and expert advice offered by well-ness. The value placed on individual experts within wellness illus-trates key attitudes towards control and trust, reinforced continu-ally within wellness media: that practices related to health should not be trusted when prescribed by the government (see: vaccines, GMOs); that managing wellness should be firmly within the hands of individuals (which may paradoxically provide a veneer of acces-sibility, until it's noted that the practices for best managing wellness remain, financially and geographically, inaccessible for the majority of people); that only other people with authentic experiences can be trusted. Frequently, personal blogs devoted to wellness will note, in "About Me" sections, that their writers are not certified nutrition-ists or medical professionals, as if their advice should be taken with a grain of salt when, ironically, this very lack of credentials is what lends them credence. Carol's doctors had no idea what was wrong with her: only others like her did.

This attitude demonstrates further aspects of the role of the per-sonal within wellness. First, just because Carol can be considered a prototype of the well body does not mean that wellness really allows for that level of sickness anymore. By placing value on the personal over the professional, wellness presupposes an absence of any serious medical condition that would require care beyond the advice of other people who have been through it. After all, the reoccurring and predominant personal narrative found in wellness media — "I left my [boring, toxic, draining] [job, city, relationship] for a new practice of [vegan, clean, whole] [baking, cooking, making], along the way healing [my autoimmune disease, my food intolerance, my child's autism]" — points to one thing, and one thing only: wellness is the best medicine.

Wellness is and is not new. There are certainly new developments and trends within wellness but some of its basic premises are long-standing. As John King wrote in the 1800s: "Although there are many maladies in which medical and medicinal treatment cannot be dispensed with, yet I am fully convinced that nearly, if not quite, one-half of the sicknesses which come under the care of medical men, could and ought to be cured solely by recourse to hygiene."[10] As old as an idea of illness as punishment is, illness as punishment for uncleanliness is perhaps even older. What is contemporary and distinctive about wellness is the nature of the uncleanliness it seeks to manage and the media through which it does so. The exposure and fear at the heart of wellness is one of a distinctively chemical and industrial nature. It is not the uncleanliness of darkness or dampness that King was most probably thinking of when he called for hygiene. The cleanliness of wellness is not about germs or infectious diseases or, really, any disease other people could probably give you. It is entirely about things that can be done to your body without your even knowing it, because the "done to" is transmitted through acts that seem perfectly innocuous, like vaccines or eating wheat. Staying clean is about avoiding things like "industrial" or "environmental": things that are directly opposed to the personal and individual. Wellness is hyper-attentive to the individual. Wellness is for you. And what benefits, beyond the physical, it can provide: "The Romantic view is that illness exacerbates consciousness. Once that illness was TB; now it is insanity...[that brings] paroxysmic enlightenment."[11] Now it is wellness.

10   Weisz, *Chronic Disease in the 20th Century*, 3.
11   Sontag, *Illness as Metaphor*, 36.

The enlightenment of wellness is directly related to the media through which it enlightens. Instead of relying solely on books, in-person meetings, support groups, or brochures distributed through doctor's offices or governmentally, as many public health campaigns, fad diets, and general health media does, wellness is accessible and participatory across many social media platforms. Instead of relying on only the publication of cookbooks, which may only be able to focus on a single dietary approach and a set number of recipes, wellness can exist through blogs, whose endless format and constant updating allows for multiple approaches (i.e. the vegan and gluten-free baking blog). Blog formats similarly allow for their authors to revise in real time as recommendations and nutritional advice shift, as seen in the years-long narrative arc of soy, once thought of as a healthy and readily available vegan source of protein but now a food to be avoided because what is readily available is only GMO. Instead of a single brochure with advice and a few images you may pick up from your doctor, wellness can exist on Instagram, which creates a daily and ongoing visual demonstration of a wellness lifestyle. Likewise, Pinterest also allows for a visually accessible and ongoing collection of wellness content. And across any platform, wellness is as easy to participate in as clicking a "pin it" button. Wellness is for you, by you.

While inextricably linked to the development of social media inasmuch as the widespread, ongoing, visually present nature of wellness would not have been fully possible prior to this media, wellness can also be linked to several other recent developments: growing awareness of climate change and the way that certain forms of media coverage of climate change make it seem, at once, like a way in which our environment is becoming toxic to us and as a set of responsibilities in consumption habits; governmental failure to contain certain things identified as toxic, both figuratively and literally, whether terrorism or lead; the local and whole food movements and, specifically, media coverage therein and the way this media has been created and adopted by both science journalism and foodies, i.e. both as science and aesthetic; the medicalization of everyday life and an increasing number of recognized conditions (to the point of beginning to distinguish between a condition, like a food intolerance, and a disease, like Celiac's); an increasing number of recognized conditions while simultaneously more and more diseases are becoming treatable, creating a catch-22 of becoming healthier and healthier while wondering what else you may have; globalization and the reoccurring discovery of uniquely healthy populations (being expressed, for example, in popularizing the "superfoods" these populations eat); the obesity epidemic and the growing belief that everything that has been popularized by both the government and fad diets is incorrect, funded by multinational corporations, and directly and solely responsible for said obesity epidemic. But, most notably, wellness can be linked directly to the rise in rates, as previously mentioned, of autism and autoimmune diseases.

In *AIDS and its Metaphors,* Susan Sontag notes that "illnesses like heart attacks and influenza that do not damage or deform the face never arouse the deepest dread."[12] Until now. There is something paradoxical about the degree of fear that is generated around autism and autoimmune diseases, because neither is (commonly) a disease that will kill you nor visually deform you. And yet wellness does generate exactly this fear. Because in a culture that values not only long-standing beliefs about self-made people but also more recent ideals about the presentation and representation of oneself, especially in the very social media in which wellness operates, these diseases represent one of the biggest contemporary fears: the inability to be oneself. Specifically the inability to *authentically* be oneself and the inability to authentically represent oneself. And furthermore, autism and autoimmune diseases represent the worst-case scenario in which this inability could happen because in both diseases *you* — whether through a body that cannot identify its cells as itself or through "the autistic brain" — are the one preventing yourself from doing so. Wellness is easier. Wellness and the "toxins" it posits as the worst imaginable sources of danger are actually much easier to admit than a problem that is, ultimately, you; a disease that is inseparable from you and who you are is worse and more difficult to imagine than a disease caused by your iPhone or wheat or GMOs. Not just difficult to imagine that a disease and its cause are one and the same as you and your body, but an outright impossibility: vaccines cause autism at an age between a few months and a few years,

12 Sontag, *Illness as Metaphor,* 128.

indicating that "the autistic brain" is not something that simply is. Everything could have been prevented. Illnesses are not things that really happen, that do not happen for any unidentifiable reason, and that do not happen to you. Wellness is the impossibility of illness. Wellness is the notion that ultimately, avoiding exposure to toxins is not enough, because the aesthetic of wellness and its practices provides a way to continually demonstrate the importance of how you are really being the best and most well and most authentic you possible. Wellness is you being your own impossibility of illness. Wellness is the best medicine.

How, then, and within this context, to understand a sick body that is comically, insanely, paradoxically, or fittingly, the most well body possible? Which is to say, through and because of illness and the specificities of what a pancreas needs, I am all of this. Having been sick long enough, cared for it long enough, and absorbed these practices of care deeply enough, this is not just a matter of practicing wellness: it is being wellness. Not a well body, necessarily. But one that is, beyond being visibly white, thin, and feminine, engaged constantly in practices of protecting-from-harm-through-ingestion. I have a low-fat, low-glycemic, low-allergen diet. I don't eat wheat, most dairy, any meat, legumes, a handful of certain fruits and vegetables, processed foods, refined or added sugar, anything that is fried; there is an obvious reason I refer to this generally as either the water diet or the nothing diet. Having done this for long enough, I am at least thirty pounds lighter than the average American woman, especially given the exercise I do daily (exercise being one of the best diabetes preventions even in an unavoidable case of pancreatic damage-induced diabetes — called Type 3, an unpopular form).

Instead of achieving and enjoying, relaxing into, the glowing well body this (should) produce, my wellness is distinctly uncomfortable. Though the well body may be the prevented body, prevention is often uncomfortable; constant perception of risk within a daily environment is uncomfortable. This, no money can adequately attend to. This, this is the only true wellness and authenticity available to the sick: the perfect appearance of ultimate health through illness. The joke is on all of us. The joke is embedded in and perpetuated through the play of privileges in different spheres. The joke is being so thin that routine surgeries, like a possible gallbladder removal, become dangerous in a body with so little room to move equipment around in, or in other procedures during which pediatric-sized equipment becomes necessary. The joke, a crueler joke, is in social moments when my eating disorder is assumed, or when it is assumed that I must enjoy and take pride in being so thin and not, in fact, see it as a sign of imminent bodily decomposition: pancreatitis is characterized by pancreatic enzymes that digest and injure surrounding tissue, essentially digesting the body itself and how else can I see weight loss except as an extension of this? This is what is authentic. This is the thin well body produced by itself. This is what you want? This is what you think looks good? Wellness may be the best medicine, but sickness is what is only, truly, for life.

Untitled (Everything is Visceral)

Mind on my Tummy

I can't remember things right now. Some things, anyway, nor can I really remember the order of things or how something began by the time I get to the end. It's my grasp that's gone, my ability to hold on and sort things out and remember the things and the sorting. Even these few sentences are getting repetitive because I can't really remember what I had been thinking to say next. This isn't the first time I've had this complete lack of grasp. The first time was when my cat died and I didn't even bother trying to read anything in English for days afterward because I couldn't remember the beginning of the sentence by the time I had gotten to the end of it (that I can remember). I'm not sad, now, and no one's dead. Now, my grasp is gone because of Amitriptyline HCL 10 mg.

Tummy on My Mind

It's not what you think. While it is true that Amitriptyline HCL 10 mg is a tricyclic antidepressant, it has a long history of off-label usage as a treatment for nerve pain or nerve damage, like nerve damage caused by a chronic illness, and the whole time my doctor was discussing the prescription and its use in relation to the gastrointestinal system with me, I couldn't tell if he was saying gastroenterology or gastroneurology.

Mind on My Tummy

It's like my gut is sad and needs antidepressants. It's like, unlike so many other people who take antidepressants for sad minds only to find themselves facing physical side effects of which weight gain and constipation are some of the most common, I, instead, am taking it for my sad gut only to find myself with mental side effects which, while not being able to remember things doesn't make me sad, exactly, do make me absolutely and completely infuriated. I can only say "it's like" because I don't have a lot of other information about sad guts, yet, and because, as an off-label usage, it is difficult to find information about Amitriptyline HCL 10 mg and nerve damage, and the whole time my doctor was saying either gastroenterology or gastroneurology, he was discussing Elavil, a version of Amitriptyline that AstraZeneca doesn't even make anymore.

Tummy on My Mind

The first step in determining whether guts can even be sad (and whether I should continue taking the Amitriptyline HCL 10 mg) is to decide what "gut" means. Because the gut is a complex system or network, including organs all the way from the salivary glands and esophagus to liver and pancreas and anus.[1] It is often characterized, within popular scientific journalism, as a computer system, a little brain or a second brain, because the enteric nervous system, which innervates the whole gut, contains every neurotransmitter that the central nervous system contains; there is nothing peripheral about it. Because there is nothing peripheral about it, the gut is also, more widely speaking, at the center of things: it may not be at the heart of the matter, but it is what runs entirely through it and because it is at the center it provides, in its own way, an answer to or model for an answer, to the question of whether my doctor was saying gastroenterology or gastroneurology, because he and I are still trying to determine what is at the center.

The enteric nervous system is extensive. It is commonly quoted that "the small intestine in humans has as many nerves as the spinal cord."[2] The gut feels. What it feels, though, is not always obvious.

---

1   Cathy Gulli, "The Brain-Gut Connection," *MacLean's* 121.45 (2008): 64–67.
2   Elizabeth Wilson, *Psychosomatic: Feminism and the Neurological Body* (Durham, NC: Duke University Press, 2004), 31.

The enteric nervous system consists of three main kinds of nerve groups, divided between two main networks (called plexuses) which serve to detect thermal, chemical, and mechanical conditions (done mainly by sensory neurons) and augment these conditions by manipulating muscle movements (like of the gut wall) and secretions (like of digestive enzymes, performed by motor neurons). Interneurons facilitate communications between sensory and motor neurons. The little or second brain labels come in because there is, relatively, little communication along the vagus nerve between the gut and the brain. The gut makes its own decisions.

As a somewhat disparate collection of organs whose main functions are best facilitated via muscle movements and secretions, who are you to make decisions of this kind? Doing so would require specific and constantly, minutely, changing information and the ability to make decisions based on this information. For instance, what is the difference between the amount of lipase and amylase, enzymes needed to break down fat and carbs, respectively, in a piece of pizza as opposed to an avocado? How do these amounts change based on the time of day or the temperature or how much water I've had to drink or what else I've eaten or how much pain I'm in or whether I've done my part properly in these decisions by taking Creon, a neatly capsuled dose of amylase and lipase? Maybe a sad gut is one that can't make decisions. Maybe a sad gut is one that hasn't been given enough information about what is at the heart of the matter. Maybe if losing my memory is enough to make me angry than being confused is enough to make my gut sad.

This confusion fits neatly into the computer model of the gut, because it depicts a network of nerves and information hubs (organs) in disarray or with crossed connections. One main aspect of the computer-gut model not often noted is how reliant this analogy is on invisibility. Because just as the stuff (hardware) that makes a computer actually compute is hidden within smooth silver surfaces, the stuff of the gut is hidden beneath skin and muscle and a rib cage and other organs. Both computers and guts rely on this invisibility to produce, continually and reliably, seamless interfaces and user interactions. "The portions of the gut innervated mainly by the enteric nervous system tend to remain outside awareness until they break down."[3] Maybe a confused gut is enough to make me sad.

Mind on My Tummy

A second model of the gut seems to refute this invisibility entirely. Instead of envisioning the gut as a computer, it can be depicted as another (more apparent) body part, that of the skin. The gut can be seen as similar to the skin because both serve as barriers, with the gut acting as "a tunnel that permits the exterior to run right through us. Paradoxically, whatever is in the lumen of the gut is thus actually outside of our bodies."[4]

The funny thing about the skin as a metaphor or model for the gut is that the skin is the largest organ humans have and the one that you never think of as being a real organ, so in some ways the gut/skin metaphor doesn't, actually, move beyond or stop relying on and reinforcing the invisibility of the gut, because it likens it to another object that seems beyond the realm of real organhood.

If the computer model of the gut serves mainly to illustrate the workings of the enteric nervous system, the skin model seems to be more so about the function of the gut (as organs rather than as nerves) as a barrier, as a thing that controls the flow of what enters and is released by our bodies, much as the skin does. Maybe having a confused gut very much on the inside of my body instead of (being able to envision it as) on the outside of my body is enough to make me sad.

Wouldn't having an external barrier within the body mean that the gut is really just a barrier to ourselves, from ourselves? Maybe being isolated is enough to make my gut sad.

Tummy on My Mind

Maybe a determination of what constitutes a sad gut doesn't need to be based on, or only on, defining what the gut, itself, is, but on whether the gut is able to experience sadness. As in, if what you are noticing is chemical, thermal, or mechanical, what about

3   Wilson, *Psychosomatic,* 37.
4   Wilson, *Psychosomatic,* 44.

this information can cause sadness? But even this question would depend on whether the gut is being defined by what it is or by what it does. Is the gut a collection of organs that do stuff or is it a bunch of nerves that decide stuff? Privileging one conceptualization over another seems to depend on another set of privileges: does your gut work or does it not work? Is your gut a thing that does things for you, that makes its own decisions, or do you have to constantly consider your gut's needs and decide, for it, what it should do and when? (Keeping in mind that any such decisions are guess work because how can you fix hardware, which inherently requires mechanical repairs, when all the hardware is inside and, anyway, what kind of hardware can be fixed just by putting more stuff, like food or Amitriptyline HCL 10 mg, into it?)

If what you are noticing is your gut's ability to notice (and regulate) mechanical, chemical, and thermal changes, what about your noticing (or what you are noticing) determines whether you want more skin or an internal computer? When your perception of an object includes "the motor adjustments we made to obtain the perception in the first place and also include[s] the emotional reactions we had then,"[5] does your perception of your gut as either a computer or as skin imply your perception of your gut as a thing you used or a thing that covers you at all times?

Mind on My Tummy

Part of the determination of whether a gut can be sad is related to the question of having either more skin or an internal computer. Because part of whether a gut can feel sad depends on how much it is yours. That is, if "ownership and agency are, likewise, related to a body at a particular instant in a particular space. The things you own are close to your body, or should be, so that they remain yours."[6] Is your gut a thing, like a computer, that you own and is inside you because through this ownership you keep it close, or is it, like skin, which is simply there with this invisible, inherent, always already embeddedness, so close to you that it is like a barrier, like

5   Antonio Damasio, *The Feeling of What Happens: Body and Emotion in the Making of Consciousness* (New York: Mariner Books, 1999), 148.
6   Damasio, *The Feeling of What Happens,* 145.

a second skin, that defies ownership because, really, how do you own your skin? Whether you own it or not matters not only for the objecthood of your gut but because this ownership is related to agency and, therefore, maintains (or consists in part of) a spatial relationship to your body, it also matters in considering whether or not your gut can be sad: are gut feelings ones that your gut has or feelings that you have or feelings that your gut gives to you? And when you stop taking Amitriptyline HCL 10 mg and find yourself much more able to write (because you are much more able to remember), now, is this satisfaction a feeling that you have or one that your gut gave you or one that you are having at the expense of your gut?

Tummy on My Mind

The question of ownership, of how you have (or feel yourself to have) your skin, and therefore the rest of your body, is at the heart of the matter of having a gut that is skin or a computer. Or, more precisely, the question is not so much one of similarity between your gut and skin or a computer, but rather a question of how differently you perceive your gut to be from the rest of your body and whether this difference (or lack thereof) is more like a computer or like skin. Meaning: if your gut is in no way dissimilar from the rest of your body, then your gut is like skin, because having a gut that is skin means having a gut that is more of the same, more of what's already there. Because your body is not, actually, a computer, having a gut that is a computer means having a gut that is different from the rest of your body.

Different in part, perhaps, because of the kind of thinking (or non-thinking) your gut does. That is, because of the kind of information the enteric nervous system pays attention to, namely mechanical, thermal, and chemical, namely not emotions, the gut as computer model is a way of encasing the gut as a data set. This encasing effects not only the gut but the way the data of the body throughout is thought of as well: if the gut is data, then data is a collection of matter and nerves and organs. Information is mass.

Information is mass and the gut is weight and this is most obviously illustrated by the fact that weight is a number, in pounds and BMI and in 10 mg being an appropriate dose of Amitriptyline HCL for a gut my size. Is the preclusion of emotional information from data based on thermal, mechanical, and chemical changes indicative of the way we think about our own emotions, the liveliness of our bodies, or the way that processing is so often portrayed as being at odds with higher level emotional thinking? Maybe being isolated is enough to make my gut sad.

Mind on My Tummy

All of these questions and the perceptual maneuvers they require are because this question of what the gut is is not one easily answered within standard considerations of embodiment. Because embodiment is so often taken to mean the way that we experience and are embodied within our physical bodies. But the question of whether the gut can be sad can't be answered entirely within such a matrix because it ultimately asks the question of how bodies, how physical matter, is embodied within us. What is it about this question that makes it so difficult to answer?

Consider, for a moment, the way that "stomach" often acts as a cipher for the entirety of the digestive system. Which, in turn, means that a word like "stomachache" can be used to mean anything from nausea to pain to hunger; it becomes not a cipher, exactly, but a way of creating opacity over physical sensations. "Stomach" is the gut/center/tunnel of the matter because a tunnel is a hole and "stomach" is a hole that indicates an inability to completely perceive and account for the complexity of the gut and I say "stomachache" even when I know the pain I'm in is in no way caused by my stomach. "Stomach" is indicative of a hole in embodiment, of a failure in perception that is similar to a kind of agnosia. Agnosia is a neurological condition in which a lack of one specific kind of sensory information (i.e. visual, auditory) prevents the recall of an object. Which, in turn, prevents a current perception of an object because how can you recognize an object if you can't remember having seen it before and how can you tell if your gut is sad if you can't even tell what your gut is or recall how it was before?

The gut is a black box that is distinct from the black box that the brain has been thought of for centuries. Because the problem of the brain's black box-ness was about an inability to access the workings of the brain based solely on physical and visual information. The problem of the black box gut is not one of mechanics but of mechanism. We know what the gut does: we put things into it and other things come out in ways that are both obvious and invisible (but not insensible). We know what the gut does but not how it decides to do those things. How does a gut determine what to shit and what to distribute? How can you have something if you don't really know what it is?

Tummy on My Mind

This question can actually be answered by a return to the gut computer model. Because it could instead be asked as: how do you own an unknown (or unknowable) product? And Apple easily answers this question: you buy it for the packaging. And, in turn, you develop that smooth shiny packaging precisely because you are aware of the unknowability of what's inside.

Mind on My Tummy

In terms of the relationship between forgetting (or an inability to remember) and an inability to recognize an object, does the fact that I stopped taking the Amitriptyline HCL 10 mg two days ago and my ability to remember is returning, somehow mean that I will or should now be better able to recognize my gut? Or, maybe, this inability only ever constitutes itself. Maybe it takes a consideration of what depression is to determine what the (sad) gut is. For example, if depression "is a breakdown not of the brain, per se, or of the liver or of the gut. It is a breakdown of the relations among organs,"[7] then maybe my gut is sad *because* I don't even know what it is.

What if my gut is sad not only because I don't know what it is, whether it is skin or a computer, but also because I never decided what it was before, before now, before I needed to, before it became sad. And maybe this confusion or inability only

7　Elizabeth Wilson, "The Work of Antidepressants: Preliminary Notes on How to Build an Alliance Between Feminism and Psychopharmacology," *Biosocieties* 1.1 (2006): 130 [125–31]; doi: 10.1017/S174585520505012X.

ever constitutes itself because consider the following excerpt from Antonio Damasio's *The Feeling of What Happens*:

> We begin with an organism made up of body proper and brain, equipped with certain forms of brain response to certain stimuli and with the ability to represent the internal states caused by reacting to stimuli and engaging repertoires of preset response. As the representations of the body grow in complexity and coordination, they come to constitute an integrated representation of the organism, a proto-self…But all of these processes — emotion, feeling and consciousness — depend for their execution on representations of the organism. Their shared essence is the body.[8]

What if something happens during the growth in complexity of bodily representations that disrupts both the complexity and ensuing coordination? What if, before you fully realize or decide what the gut is, you are taught (if that's the right word) that this decision is meaningless or unnecessary because your gut is just a thing you have or a thing you use and what is complex about that? What if the disruption to complexity is the utter simplicity of the gut-computer and gut-skin models? What if the development of complexity or coordination is on some level related to other neurological development, like growing up, and you have been sick since you turned 18? What if these disruptions to complexity, because they create an inability to depict accurate representations of the body, further inhibit coordination because you cannot communicate nothing, or, you can, only this means the communication of confusion. What if this series of disruptions creates a situation of alienation, wherein the gut is neither a skin nor a computer but a different actualization of the gut being external, in that it has become external to the knowing self. And, therefore, because it is within me but without me, the gut has no choice but to have its own feelings.

Tummy on My Mind

And, now, what kind of interruption to complexity and coordination is going on when my stomach hurts to the point that it is

8   Damasio, *The Feeling of What Happens,* 248.

distracting and I can barely focus on what I'm reading, let alone write anything? It's a deceptive interruption because in this situation it only seems like the simplicity of my stomachache is interrupting the complexity of my thinking, because, really, what is going on is a series of disruptions: the simplicity of the pain of my body, followed by an immediate awareness that even as I say "stomachache" I know that it's not my stomach, so if it's not my stomach then what is it, and if I don't know what it is, really, today, then how can I do anything about it, and if I can't even think straight, now, is this better or worse than not being able to remember anything?

I'm too distracted by this simple pain to continue being able to focus on questions of the embodiment of the gut, so perhaps it's time to fully, actually, consider sadness now and leave the gut at this: it's a hole, like a tunnel, but not empty. If it's a lack, as a hole, that's only because it's a lack of awareness; as a body part for which there is no complete awareness, the gut exists in a state of unembodiment. This isn't the same as disembodiment because the problem is not one of detachment. Rather, the gut is within and without and we are within and without the gut as well.

Mind on My Tummy

So, depression. Allowing for a standard hierarchy of complexity within emotions, it would perhaps be prudent to start with a definition of sadness, as feelings of sadness are the building blocks of depression. In fact, by some accounts, depression is simply sustained feelings of sadness. This continuity of feeling, regardless of other criteria, is always a part of determining (or diagnosing) depression. In turn, this linking of diagnosis and defining raises the question of whether depression can be defined in a way that differentiates depression as only ever active (as in actual) when it is a thing a person is doing from depression as a state separate from a standardized enactment of that state. Or, is there a core quality or state of depression that can be identified through its isolation from the set of symptoms that arises in being depressed? If so, it would seem to be this core depression that the gut is capable of because how can a gut exhibit other behaviors associated with depression like not getting out of bed and substance abuse, and I wonder if it is harder or easier to diagnose depression in a person than it is to diagnose a physical illness in a gut. The statistics would seem to indicate it's easier, on the basis that psychiatric medications are some of the most widely prescribed, and I have been sick for years with, in part, the condition of being in a diagnostic "no man's land," to quote the same doctor who said either gastroenterology or gastroneurology while providing me with an unpopular usage of a popular drug and I do understand that this is not exactly a one-to-one comparison but how much easier is it for you to think of and know a time when you felt sad than it is to identify, locate, and define what, exactly, your pancreas does?

Tummy on My Mind

My simply painful gut is distracting me again.

Mind on My Tummy

Given the frequency with which gastrointestinal symptoms are reported by people with clinical depression, namely changes to appetite and weight, to the degree that such symptoms are part of the criteria for a diagnosis of depression, it may seem like a sad gut is really just a similar psychosomatic state. But the way that physical symptoms arise in depression is such that they are as a result of an existing emotional state. Which, yes, as a set of neurological characteristics is itself definitely physical, but the point being that the entire concept of psychosomatic illness is based on the idea that the body is entirely under the influence of the mind. A sad gut, a gut that is its own physical symptom generator, as in a gut that is already sick, is not producing these symptoms as a result of existing emotions. This in turn gives rise to two questions: one, what to call or how to consider this kind of anti-psychosomatic or psychosomatic resistant sadness, and, two, addressing the kind of internal anthropomorphism at play here.

It's an anthropomorphism inherent in the term "sad gut" because a gut is not a person and a person is the only thing that gets sad. Many body parts, though, are subject to this kind of anthropomorphism: the heart's (or penis') mind of its own, for example. This kind of part–whole anthropomorphism, wherein a part of us, because it's us, must therefore be comparable to or simply a smaller model of the whole of us, is useful to our discussion here, but limited by its unidirectional nature. First, it does provide an existing understandable model through which to think sometimes unintelligible or unknown questions. However, part–whole anthropomorphism fails to take into account how the whole may be, actually, comparable to or a larger model of its part, how, maybe, anthropomorphizing the gut only ever further reinforces a failure in understanding the gut and how much it constitutes us.

Tummy on My Mind

Even when trying to define sadness, its location in the gut (as opposed to "us" or the brain) means that it is always in relation to a physical sensation. Despite that oft-cited figure meant to illustrate the sensitivity of the gut, what it is capable of being sensitive to is still defined narrowly and physically. Can an organ (especially one which is not one, but many) have a feeling that is more than the physical feeling of pain? (Is pain only physical, ever?) More of a feeling meaning exactly that, a feeling that is more like an emotion than a physical sensation. Is it that the physical pain of a sick gut becomes, over time or through interpretation or through interpretation over time, a feeling of sadness?

Sometimes I feel pain but I don't also feel sick and sometimes I feel sick but I'm not in pain but whether I'm in pain or feeling sick or feeling neither, there is always the physical presence of sickness. There is always a sick gut. There is no clear causation, no psychosomatic linking between psychological emotions and physical symptoms, or things that happen that become symptoms, or things that are felt that become symptoms, because, in this already sick saddened gut, the sheer force of physical fact overrides any attempts at separating the physical from the emotional; pain is pain is sadness is sickness is the gut. Saying that sad guts are always also sick guts doesn't mean that the sadness is being caused by the sickness, because not all sick guts will be sad and because here, in the gut, sickness and sadness are one and the same. Saying that sad guts are always also sick guts isn't the same as saying that sick people are always also sad, but that certain physical sensations within sickness are always also emotions. Emotions that organs are having. Consider again the diagnostic criteria for depression set out in the DSM-IV, and the inclusion there of items like changes to behavior or loss of interest in prior activities, and, alongside this, consider symptoms of a gastrointestinal illness like ulcerative colitis or Crohn's, which can include alternating diarrhea and constipation, and bloating and nausea and bleeding. Alternating diarrhea and constipation are nothing if not a change in behavior. A sad gut is one that no longer wants to do what it (maybe) used to do. A sad gut is one that can no longer remember how to do what it used to do. A sad gut, in this not remembering and not desiring (because it doesn't know what to desire anymore) recognizes that sadness is the absence of information. A sad gut, knowing that information is mass, concurrently recognizes that the absence of information has direct physical effects. In this sad gut, alternating diarrhea and constipation become a mechanism for the regulation of or searching for information: holding onto, letting it all out, trying to communicate. Because sadness, any emotion, is not just about having the capacity to feel the emotion but also the ability to communicate it. A sad gut is one that is trying to tell you something.

Upset Stomach

If the gut is a hole in embodiment, and if sadness, or at least the sadness of guts, is a lack of knowledge or information, then these states lead to a third condition of misunderstanding because of too little information: what if I never tell you how it feels? What if, throughout this whole discussion of guts and sadness, I never tell you how my gut feels and all that is really felt, here, is how unfelt, how unembodied, the gut is? Because I can say "pain" and "stomachache" over and over, but what do you actually know? But this is, in a similar but slightly different way, exactly how my gut feels: I feel what I don't know. I feel, exactly, what I don't know how to feel, as in how to interpret, except that, also, at the same time, my gut hurts almost all the time and also, at the same time, I know exactly that something is wrong and the core of this feeling is more correct than any specific information (diagnosis, pancreatic physiology) can ever be. This is part of what I mean when I say psychosomatic-resistant, in that it is simultaneously, always, both of these feelings, and there is never really one without the other, and (after years of this shit) it no longer matters which is causing the other. This is why, in part, continuity is such a main part of the diagnostic criteria for depression: it no longer matters why but *that*; that it continues; that the gut is a hole, but like a tunnel. Continuity is also important in diagnosing depression because it helps to distinguish between sadness that is related to individual life events and that passes, as expected, and sadness that persists, with or without apparent external causes. But how do you know what's expected? How can you determine what sadness is if there is no standardized or reliable baseline? Because, maybe, not knowing a baseline, non-sad, gut feeling means that I'm constantly mis-feeling, miscommunicating with my gut. All I remember from before, from before I was sick, was never feeling anything, never knowing, and I still don't know (that much) now, even though I feel all the time. Maybe this is actually how it's supposed to feel. Maybe the psychosomatic resistance is all in my head and I've begun to think that maybe everyone feels like this, like this is what digestion is supposed to, normally, feel like, and I'm just feeling it wrong. But I've been asking, especially after meals shared with family or friends, and it seems like not everyone else is in pain most of the time, though this doesn't entirely clear up the issue of whether what I'm feeling as pain is, actually, being correctly interpreted as such; maybe everyone else feels what I feel but their guts don't hurt. And then I was watching television with my parents and we were interrupted (or the show was) by a commercial for Victoza™, a blood sugar-regulating drug, a pancreas-regulating drug, and the commercial, as mandated by law, told us that pancreatitis, a side effect, may be fatal and you may have the worst stomach pain you've ever felt (maybe they didn't say that exactly) that may extend through your back, with or without vomiting, and we were interrupted. What if no one ever tells me how it is supposed to feel?

Mind on My Tummy

This interruption may be telling. Because what it illustrates is the way that a sad (sick) gut makes itself felt and present, or at least one way that it can do this: as an interruption to normal communication, as a break, like a commercial, but one that communicates side effects. Remembering that the key aspect of the gut as skin metaphor was the way that the gut came to function as a place of interaction between the inside and outside of the body, consider the following description of Andrew Solomon's depression, mainly the way he dealt with it: "Largely unable to feel or connect with others, Solomon is able to enter into a relation of reciprocated care with his father through the gut."[9] Meaning that Solomon, through having meals prepared for and fed to him by his father, is able to find enough support in this relationship to ultimately further his recovery from clinical depression. This would make sense given, again, that the gut is "a vital organ in the maintenance of relations to others."[10] The gut is about communication, as a conduit (or barrier) for the weight of information, and if sadness is the lack of information, then this lack disrupts communication between what two things, exactly? It doesn't have to be more complicated than to say that the sadness of the gut interrupts internal to external, and vice versa, communications: it makes obvious the lack of clarity, the lack of information, between what is apparent and what is in the hole running through what is apparent.

Upset Stomach

Even as I'm writing this, trying to communicate, what I am mostly thinking about (being distracted by) is the way that the pain I'm feeling now (a slight departure from, more urgent than, the pain I usually feel) how it feels almost like hunger pangs except that instead of emptiness I feel a tunneling. And I am still wondering if, maybe, it really could be just hunger pangs. Wouldn't it be easier if my gut was just irritable instead of sad? Wouldn't it be easier if I could fully join the IBS masses instead of that pancreatitis interruption which may be fatal? How do I know it's not just IBS? Even when I am told this is also what it is, under every hypothetical model of IBS, having had acute pancreatitis or having chronic pancreatitis creates the physiological changes thought to be responsible for causing IBS — is this really two diseases, one larger one, or two insurance billing codes? How do you know what a disease is supposed to feel like?

Maybe the memory loss caused by the Amitriptyline HCL 10 mg was never a side effect but a desired and desirable main effect, so that this whole time I could have been forgetting how sad my gut is.

9   Wilson, *Psychosomatic,* 47.
10   Wilson, *Psychosomatic,* 45.

Mind on My Tummy (Again, Differently)

Maybe it would be even easier if there was nothing to remember. Maybe biology is just that scary and the answer to fear like this is to frame ideas like those being articulated here as just trafficking too heavily in biology and biological determinism and the attributing of agency to things that are just things as not only poor (queer, feminist) scholarship, but as trivial. See: "Discussion of the biological causes of depression might be plausible, but I find them trivial. I want to know what environmental, social, and familial factors trigger those biological responses — that's where things get interesting."[11] Because it is only within the environmental, social or familial that "things" are interesting? Because the body (as in, biology, not as in the Body) is boring? Because it seems like the problem is not as much one of biological determinism as it is one of biological predeterminism, because the problem is not one of how your body is now but of the (seeming) impossibility (or at least intense undesirability) of your body, as it was or always has been or (probably) always will be, biologically, determining you, or (more threateningly) determining your fate. Biologically predetermined as in, your body, a physical form, existed before you were conscious of it (or conscious at all).

I wasn't born this way, actually; shit happens.

This biological predeterminism is such a problem because, if true, it would mean that "you" are not better than your body. It would mean being unable to think your way out of a physical form. Not only think your way out of it, but the mind–body separation that is necessarily maintained by a struggle against biological predeterminism means thinking you can overcome your body.

I can't. (And would I really want to? That would be a lot of effort, for what? Not more life, really, nor even, probably, a more intellectually satisfying one. One less filled with shit? Maybe.)

And, as a side note, how can you find biological relations to depression trivial after, as Cvetkovich writes, having just witnessed multiple friends die of AIDS?

---

11 Ann Cvetkovich, *Depression: A Public Feeling* (Durham, NC: Duke University Press, 2012), 15.

Full of Shit

Maybe there is something biologically predetermined about the gut that leaves it susceptible to depression. Like the fact that it handles shit all day. The constant presence of or continuous engagement in the process of making shit opens space for another gut–brain connection or point of similarity. Within neuroscience, and the way that neuroscience is written or rewritten within critical theory, the main process that the brain is engaged in and which effects all further possibilities and processes of engagement is plasticity. That is, the brain, like a computer, is open to the reworking of neural networks, the formation of new connections, forged through patterns of behavior and information input, that produce both positive and negative change; plasticity is the quality that allows for everything from the learning of new behaviors to the formation of habits to the personality changes that may come from brain injuries. Everything the brain does is related to plasticity, however circuitously. Because the gut is always full of shit and all behaviors and processes that happen within it are tied to this fundamental engagement, a relationship can be drawn wherein the brain is to plasticity as the gut is to shit. Much as plasticity is the main vehicle for change in the brain, shit is for the gut. Because shit is entirely about repetition with difference. Plasticity is about being open to change, whether positive or negative, through inscription and reinscription. The shitty plasticity of the gut is about repetition as opposed to inscription because inscription implies a continuous or constantly present surface on which things happen, being erased or laid over one another, whereas shit is entirely gotten rid of and started anew; it is both continuous and begins and ends and begins all the time; shit allows for newness (and ongoingness) over habit. Shit is not habit-forming because its main purpose is to find the best in things, to sort through what could go into it and save those things most useful, passing them on; plasticity more or less has to take what it is given, developing habits that may be ultimately harmful or losing traits that were useful. It's not that shit is above malfunction, either, but even in times of alternating diarrhea and constipation, shit is happening.

Shitty plasticity trivializes mind–body separations. Shitty plasticity trivializes notions of biological responses triggered by a you that is (somehow) separate from your shit(-producing gut). Shitty plasticity illustrates the way that, because determining what is needed from what should become shit requires an orchestrated series of actions across multiple organs, across multiple kinds of cells, even including non-human microbes which reside in the gut, this is more than a reaction. A reaction is a simple mechanism, like an unstoppable Rube Goldberg machine. Shitty plasticity requires communicative decision-making. And emotional variation as well: imagine the difference between the way that intestinal eukaryotic cells must communicate with non-human microbes versus the way that the pancreatic cells negotiate differences in function between endocrine and exocrine portions of the organ. Finding biologically oriented gut–brain or mind–body connections trivial turns all of this into an extended metaphor, but remembering the way that the gut is like barrier or conduit to the outside world means that none of this communication is hypothetical.

The looming specter of the constant reinforcement of the importance and supremacy of the social, environmental, and familial over the biological within critical theory creates the condition of theoretical determinism.

Upset Stomach

I find environmental, social, and familial conditions that may be contributing to my being sick plausible, but trivial, because my doctor and I are no longer, and haven't been for years, looking for why I got sick in the first place but why I continue to be. As in, it no longer matters why, but that. Like depression.

I cried twice this week. The timing seemed off, because earlier in the week, for days, I was in enough pain that I should have gone to the emergency room, but didn't, and it was only a day or two after, after I was already feeling better, that I started crying. Maybe, like shit, it takes some time to come to the surface. Maybe I wouldn't have cried if I was still taking the Amitriptyline HCL 10 mg. Maybe if I wasn't in the face of others' perceptions of the trivialness of my gut, I wouldn't be feeling so defensive, so sad, on behalf of my sad gut.

Full of Shit

Being full of shit, both in the way that the gut is and as an idiomatic expression, is about disbelief. Which is also a reoccurring theme within neuroscience and popular narratives therein, namely the "epistemic shock that is said to accompany trauma."[12] Earlier I felt conflicted in my decisions to link or not link being sick and being sad, for the way such linking often contributes to reinforcing the presence of epistemic shock after trauma as the (only) appropriate or accurate response. But what if it's not that the trauma of being sick has caused me to disbelieve my own (perception of) my gut but that the trauma of realizing how little I (am able to) know about my gut causes me to disbelieve that any of this shit could be trivial?

Upset Stomach

A large part of Ann Cvetkovich's project in *Depression* is to open up the idea that depression is firmly within and constituted by the everyday and the ordinary, a linking that has been taken up and reinforced by many queer theorists' considerations of queer depression or queer melancholic affect. The thing about Cvetkovich's efforts in particular is the way that the ordinary and everyday are often, overtly or not, linked to the insignificant (and trivial): for example, her description of "what seemed like ordinary or insignificant activities — going swimming, doing yoga, getting a cat, visiting a sick friend."[13]

Having a sad gut that is in pain almost all the time means that it is never clear what within the everyday is ordinary or trivial or insignificant and sometimes, like shit, you only know after the fact.

Dead Serious

Even while I'm full of shit, I'm also dead serious. I'm not joking. I take shit seriously. Just because it's something that seems commonplace, just because you may not want or need to talk about it (when it happens), just because this may seem like an extended joke

12 Cvetkovich, *Depression,* 1.
13 Cvetkovich, *Depression,* 82.

aimed at the shittiness of (some) queer/feminist theory, some jokes kill me. Because what is at stake here, and what is being changed by the work going on here, is my body. Really, physically. This is not theoretical. As much as it may speak to taboos or being anal there is, simultaneously, nothing theoretical about shit. Shit is a fact of life, which is what I mean when I say "shit happens."

I'm interested in shit and the processes of shitty plasticity it facilitates precisely because it happens every day; it leaves open the most opportunities for gut–brain communication because, as we saw in Andrew Solomon's negotiation of depression via communication, through the gut with his father, sometimes the answer to sadness is not a "cure," but to do exactly that: answer it, communicate with it, including any and all internal varieties. This could be made even clearer through my Amitriptyline HCL 10 mg, because the mechanism at work there was one that dealt directly with the communication between gut nerves and brain nerves, disrupting this pathway in an attempt to stop pain. Maybe this disruption was why Amitriptyline didn't fully work for me; while it did stop (some of) the pain, it failed to provide the communication and information my sad gut sorely needs.

Full of Shit

Maybe it's unfair to trivialize Cvetkovich's "trivial." Maybe it's unfair because what if a perception of triviality was not a matter of opinion but of experience? As in, maybe Cvetkovich (or others who are firmly in a certain anti-biological determinism camp) just hasn't experienced the kind of necessity that makes apparent what is and isn't trivial. What if before you decide what your gut is it's clear that this decision is meaningless or unnecessary and, therefore, trivial, so that by extension, the gut itself is trivial as a lack of unnecessary information? What if the gut de-trivializes itself, makes itself apparent, through the only mechanisms it really has access to, namely shit and nerves, and therefore through pain and upset stomachs and alternating diarrhea and constipation? What if the comedian Tig Notaro was somehow right when she says that maybe (just maybe) it was all those jokes she made for years about her small breasts that came to result in her breast cancer? What if the sadness of the gut is purely a product of its taken-for-granted-ness, which has resulted in a lack of information (which no longer seems trivial) that has been shaped by forces of the everyday, the insignificant, the apparently unnecessary?

How do you learn to pay attention?

Maybe my doctor would know better. Maybe it's called "medical attention" for a reason. Because that's also about paying for and getting a kind of attention specific to a part you may not know. But medical attention is an oddly circuitous route of perception that is more like a Mobius strip than a straightforward relationship between two separate things. See: a definition of disease as "something which always speaks a language that is at one in its existence and its meaning with the gaze that deciphers it...a language inseparably read and reading."[14] Medical attention constitutes itself. Disease, to follow Foucault, via its signs and symptoms, communicates its presence to the medical gaze that is, simultaneously, always already seeing disease. What if this same logic applies to the relationship between you and your gut, but in an even more pronounced way? Because in the case of the medical gaze it can be said that, physically, signs (as original, real, signs of symptoms) exist indicating the presence of disease before or regardless of the medical gaze; the medical gaze validates this presence, validates the disease, and constitutes it as such, but it does not (usually) (always) do this in the absence of an original sign. Meaning, there is always already a presence of a physical sign before there is also a gaze; there is an order of events that describes the way medical attention becomes a relationship between two things, between the sign and the gaze; what medical attention truly constitutes are symptoms. But, now, consider the kind of attention you can give your gut: there are no two separate things. In order for you to be a you capable of paying attention, you have to be a you in a body capable of sustaining the physical functions necessary for, in turn, sustaining that attention. You are your gut. It can be shitty. The attention you can give your gut is a form of inseparability. Like the gut is a hole, like a tunnel, but not empty, that is inside and outside at once. Like the gut is a hole, but not empty, heard in a language that is being generated and understood simultaneously, a language "read and reading." Read and reading as

14 Michel Foucault, *The Birth of the Clinic: An Archaeology of Medical Perception,* trans. Alan Sheridan Smith (London: Routledge, 2003), 96.

in a form of attention that is both ongoing and already happened (but not over). What if before you need to or knew you would need to, you decided that the gut is either a thing you use or a thing you have, and now, having read it (but not understood) it is difficult to keep reading?

The applicability of Foucault's consideration of the medical gaze to the kind of gaze and attention possible within oneself, as constituting and constituted by, illustrates an important point to which we will return, later. Namely, that given the physicality inherent in both the medical gaze and the gaze you can give yourself, while maintaining distinctions between the two, it is clear that the medical model is not nor should it stand as the only (or, as a cipher for) the entire concepts of "biology" or "physical."

Maybe my gut is already engaged in processes of being read and reading, even if only through the seemingly non-narrative information of chemical, mechanical and thermal changes. Maybe my sad gut is better at paying attention because it's sad. This is not wishful thinking or unfounded. Because depression is a problem for philosophers and neuroscientists and cognitive psychologists beyond the situation I am articulating here. Because why would depression have evolved? Given that there are accounts of depression and different kinds of melancholy dating back to premodern times, why would evolution select for traits or personality features prone to developing depression? What beneficial purpose could depression serve?

Maybe it's about attention. Maybe being sad means being able to pay attention better. Maybe "the anatomy of focus is inseparable from the anatomy of melancholy."[15] The thinking behind this hypothesis is as follows: being depressed triggers processes of introspection, specifically concerning situations that may have given rise to said depression, and that this increased analytical concentration serves to, ultimately, help people find paths out of negative situations. While obviously such an effect does not cancel out the loss of life that clinical depression is responsible for, this doesn't mean that there is not something useful to take from this, for sad guts. Because

15 Andrew Solomon, "The Anatomy of Melancholy," *The New Yorker,* January 12, 1998, 48, http://www.newyorker.com/magazine/1998/01/12/ anatomy-of-melancholy.

multiple studies have shown that this increased introspection does, indeed, increase analytical capabilities in depressed persons, to the extent that such introspection is included in diagnostic criteria. The term for such an increased introspection is rumination.

All the gut does is ruminate. Rumination is digestion. Rumination is the reason that children put things in their mouths in order to know them; because it is perhaps implicitly understood, before it is understood that the gut must be either a thing you use or a thing you have, that ingesting an object is critical to understanding. Rumination is a simultaneously physical and cognitive process. Consciousness has physical effects; thought and attention are physical processes; why should this process not take place within a space, like the gut, that has the capacity for endless input and output? Shitty plasticity and unending repetition allow for the temporal differences that rumination may create, the gaps between input and output, or the kind of attention spent on one but not the other. Like that fact that I only took Amitriptyline HCL 10 mg (and it was only 10 mg) for one week but I have spent the past month still with it, here.

Upset Stomach

Who knows better what acceptance means, me or my gut? On the one hand, I understand enough to feel that being in pain every day is actually preferable to being in pain and constantly trying to get better, especially in the face of medical and personal understanding of words like "progress" and "chronic;" because at least just being in pain isn't disappointing. On the other hand, what is remarkable about this sick gut is the way that there are many ways it could perform badly, be hindered by a couple bad parts, but shitty plasticity allows for the fact that my gut is still doing things, a lot of things, comparably pretty well. What is adaptation if not a form of acceptance?

As rumination is shaped by physical processes of the gut and shitty plasticity, it both relies on and creates a state of flow. By flow I don't mean flow like being in the zone, like being in a state of easy, fluid attention. By flow I do mean that rumination is about movement, specifically the movement of the gut–brain space, which moves things and is moving. By flow I mean the movement surrounding and generated by things that have the quality of fluidity. Things that are viscous. Like organs. Like the gut, where everything is visceral.

Visceral, meaning having the qualities of viscera; meaning organs, usually the gut; meaning organs usually in the center; meaning the organs that take up and make up the majority of the space often called the body cavity. Visceral, as in having to do with the center of things. Visceral, as in having to do with the center of the body.

So what if I never tell you how it feels? So what if all I can do is try to say the same thing to you as I say to myself over and over? So what if all I do is say things (maybe the same thing) over and over? So what if over and over is the clearest thing I can tell you about how it feels?

I think you probably already know: the statistics are in my favor. Take, for example, the fact that out of a sample group of fifteen coworkers, expanded slightly to include immediate family members: one has rheumatoid arthritis, one is in remission from lung cancer, one has skin cancer, one has a pancreatic disease, one has a brother dead of brain cancer, one has parents dead (one sudden, young, one of old age), one has a son dead in an accident, one is caring for a mother-in-law with colon cancer (stage IV, advanced, the same one herself in remission from lung cancer). I think you maybe already know. I could go on: one has a father dead, recently, of unknown cause but not old age, one has a mother with double hip replacements, one has an uncle in remission from colon cancer, one has a close family friend with MS. So what if I never tell you how it feels?

These are not things I've remembered as much as things I'm coming to realize, or coming to realize that I already knew, too. First, again, rumination is a physical process. Because of this, and because rumination is a way to name both digestion and thinking, rumination and (especially) attending to rumination via practices of attention is about accumulation and absorption. It is a process of becoming through absorption. Because the gut is either like the skin, like a permeable barrier, or like a computer, like a thing with multiple interfaces, or like a hole, like a tunnel, like a space, full of shit: the gut is about accumulation and the absorption of accumulated materials through rumination.

Gut Feelings

When I said "everything is visceral" what I meant was that there is the potential for visceral moments everywhere. I meant that the sample group of coworkers are people both involved in their own visceral moments and capable of producing ones I experience. When I said that one of my coworkers has skin cancer what I didn't say was that he also has a six-month-old baby at home and I feel this, viscerally, within the possibilities inherent in my own body and in some ways I feel the six-month-old to be within my own bodily possibilities as well.

The accumulation (through a capacity for sensitivity inherent in the gut, through the way the gut is innervated, literally given nerves, throughout) of visceral moments is the process of becoming a visceralized body. Even as I'm remembering things, a few things, now, I'm not quite sure what to do with these things, how to tell you. Because this is simultaneously the easiest and hardest thing I've had to learn and it is difficult to articulate because it has been characterized not by a series of articulated realizations but by a series of disarticulations. Such that when I say "the visceralized body is the body in a state of accumulating visceral moments," I am also meaning to say that the visceral is striking, as in being caught in (by) the gut, as in you feel it being caught, as in maybe this hurts, as in how do you dislodge an object caught in the inside of your body, as in how do you dislodge an object that is really a feeling from the inside of your body, as in maybe this hurts, as in there's no feeling better because how do you dislodge a feeling that's really an organ from the inside of your body, as in maybe you already know how this feels (and maybe you don't): visceral as in a collection of organs that create the body cavity, as in the viscous qualities (related to movement, and therefore space and time) of these organs, as in the things that organs are capable of feeling and being made felt. Visceral as in bodies having feelings. Visceral as in bodies making themselves felt.

The Visceralized Body

The visceralized body is the result of the accumulation of visceral moments, accumulated through the body and specifically through the gut, because the gut is entirely about absorption. Because the gut is a hole, like a tunnel, it not only is space but creates a path to the brain through rumination: a term for the kind of absorption the gut performs and the process of becoming, through digestion and thinking, this describes.

Even as I don't know what my gut is, even as sadness is the lack of information in the face of need, the information I need now is not a definition of nor even a definitive perception of my gut. Because I know what I do sense and I know that my gut is sad and that this sadness is like a hole, but not empty. I just need to know how else it could feel. I do and do not need you to tell me how it feels (because you probably don't know either, because is your gut like a skin or like a computer? You know). Because nerve endings do not in and of themselves create feelings, information (even a lot of it) is not the same as meaning. But what information (especially a lot of it) can provide is context.

Because a cavity is a hole, like a hollow, a body cavity, it is also a kind of decay: a relational kind of decay in which decay is a product of the relationship between your teeth and the bacteria in your mouth. In the visceralized body, this can become a kind of decay that is a product of a relationship between your body and lack of information that comes to constitute and decay the relationship between you and your body. (Even as I'm writing "you" and separately "your body," I wish I wasn't. It still feels somewhat true. At the same time, I am my body and my body is me and maybe this is a kind of acceptance that my gut and I can both come to and practice together — only together.)

If you don't know how this feels, and I don't know if you do, this may be because the inside of the body is a philosophically-historically inaccessible place, as Drew Leder writes it in *The Absent Body,* wherein "a viscous [internal organ] is largely irreversible with corporeal foci. It cannot be summoned up for personal use, it cannot be turned ecstatically upon the world. It's recessiveness is not simply a function of a current gestalt but of an innate resistance."[16]

Really? Tell that to my sad gut. (Asshole).

"Innate resistance" only in an able body. "Ecstatically" being ideal or possible only in an able body. "Irreversible" only in an able body

16 Drew Leder, *The Absent Body* (Chicago, IL: University of Chicago Press, 1990), 54.

not full of shit, continually reversing and releasing. "Recessiveness" only when your gut is only ever a thing you use or a thing you have. "Innate" only when you do not care about this recessiveness; "innate" only when you do not have to care.

Or, in a visceralized body, there is no "turned ecstatically upon" because the gut, like a barrier, like a tunnel, like the skin, is already the inside and outside at once. In a visceralized body, there is no "turned ecstatically upon" unless you consider shitting (or any other form of profuseness and excessiveness) ecstatic. This, even just saying (being able to say) "visceralized body" is a "turned ecstatically upon." In a visceralized body, there is no "innate resistance" (to attention) because innate resistance to corporeal foci is only possible when there's nothing to pay attention to. In the visceralized body, there is everything to pay attention to. "Innate resistance" is, really, a misnomer for what is really the most basic and intense privilege of the able body: there is no resistance if there is no need.

The relational quality of the decay at the cavity of the visceralized body extends to an overall externally relational quality as well. The visceralized body is not just about the inside of your own body. In part because the experience of visceral moments includes moments where other bodies make your own body felt, differently. As in my coworker with cancer and a baby; I feel all of this, though differently, of course, than he does. Not only because I am removed from the pragmatics and the daily experience of it but because all I am ultimately feeling is still my own body: within the context of the information of his. Visceralized bodies, characterized as they are by a simultaneously internal–external, relational body cavity, are open to each other. Secondly, being so open, visceralized bodies provide room for feeling the things you don't have. For instance, consider the term HIV–. Because information is mass, an absence of information about one's own body and especially information that is or is not determined to be absent in relation to others' is also a state that can be viscerally felt.

This capacity of the visceralized body, its ability to make itself felt, its felt-ness, can also be put another way: even with centuries devoted to the development of medical imaging and auditory technologies for surveying the inside of the body, the stomach (and other visceral organs, the intestines) is still an organ you can hear clearly with only your own ears. You can also hear other people's, clearly, with only your own ears.

The "innate resistance" that characterizes the able body and Leder's body is ultimately irrelevant to the visceralized body because it's sickness that begins to diminish any notion of "innate." It's sickness that both causes the accumulation of visceral moments and causes the moments themselves; it's sickness that creates the need that changes a lack of information into such a need, that changes "innate" perceptions only when you become suddenly aware of how much you can't perceive and why can't you — and would I feel better if I could?

Maybe a resistance that can be found or felt in the visceralized body is one not about the body itself but of a resistance to resisting: a resistance to getting better, in certain ways, to becoming un- or de-visceralized. Because it's (almost) easier to be in pain every day than it is to be in pain and try constantly not to be. Because at least in pain, you know how you feel. Because the visceralized body isn't looking for context that would inform a way out.

Talking about being sick in this way, linking sickness to a visceralized body, is an obstacle for me here and one I'm hesitant to address head on. Because it is one thing to say that sickness can cause visceral moments; it is another to say, or to imply, or to write a definition, that all visceral bodies must be sick. As if there were nothing else visceral to experience. On the other hand, I feel and know these things through and because of a body that is sick at the center, at the gut; I have a gastrointestinal disease characterized in part by malnutrition. Everything I ingest and absorb passes through this, is fully absorbed and passed on or not. Everything else within my body becomes, because of this. The pain, too, travels, encompasses my stomach and back and sides, changes my posture; changes the movements that become available to me. Everything is visceral. And I remember enough from before this happened to know that it is only like this now because of being sick.

And perhaps I shouldn't worry about defining visceral through sickness because as my sample group shows, there are already plenty here with me.

And in these moments, with others, I do not really mean "moment" as a singular event but as an ongoing time. As in: there was the moment I found out my coworker has cancer, the moment I remembered that he had a baby, the moment I went home and told my partner about this, as if it were one moment, and the moment after that when I said I was still thinking about it. And, now, much later, when I continue to think it and write it here.

Shit is continuously beginning and ending.

What an ongoing visceral moment includes is the ability for the visceralized body to attend to its possibilities as well as to its present. On the one hand, "my future is written in my body," and at the same time, "I am not writing a will or medical report."[17]

What does so much absorption produce? Consumption? Consumption as in all-consuming, but not totalizing. As in, just as the gut constitutes the body through digestion, consuming can include the way the gut can take of even as it is adding to. Because the gut is a hole, like a cavity, and because cavities must always include a relationship between at least two things, and because everything can go in either direction in a gut, the gut can begin to produce a decay through too much absorption as well, not only not enough: the gut can absorb so much it begins to absorb, to consume, the rest of the body. In one way, the gut becomes consuming when, in a visceral moment, I find that I've lost weight between doctors' appointments, despite no changes to diet or exercise; having failed to absorb everything else I've put in it, the gut must turn to the rest of my body. In another way, the gut demonstrates its ability to be consuming every time I'm unable to pay attention to the thing at hand. Every day, whether I always realize it or not, my gut consumes my attention. This dual absorbing–consuming quality of visceralized bodies, their guts, makes clear a key aspect about a relationship of decay: while I can decide what goes into my gut, I cannot control what comes out of it nor can I control what it decides to take. A centralized sense of agency, like a brain, like a computer, like a body that doesn't have parts to which a sense of autonomy are always attributed, like a body that probably doesn't have a heart with a mind of its own, like an able body, is lacking. Nothing is centralized in a visceralized body. Especially agency, because even though the gut is a tunnel, like a hole, in the center, it is also internal and external simultaneously.

17 Anne Boyer, "Not Writing," *The Poetry Foundation,* 2015, https://www.poetryfoundation.org/poems-and-poets/poems/detail/58316.

I am not very apologetic about saying things like "Tell that to my sad gut. (Asshole)," because by saying things like that I am also already beginning to articulate a theoretical-political position occupied by the visceralized body. Because it's not, it can't be, only about how it feels. Because what do you do with how it feels? Because a visceralized body is open to others and what do you do when you find that so few are open to yours? Because the personal is political, right? Because what is more personal than shit? Because, for instance, when I tell my partner about the weight loss, how it's tied to shit and being sick, am I not only forging a new openness between bodies but simultaneously occupying a political position that argues for exactly a kind of unapologetic nature that runs counter to existing sexist and heteronormative constructions of femininity (i.e. a feminine body that never shits, let alone tells a partner about it)? Because the visceral is political, right?

Furthermore, by saying things like "Tell that to my sad gut. (Asshole)," and thereby continually reinforcing the feelings my organs are having, by attending to those feelings, and by depicting a body wherein attention and therefore agency is a force subject to both absorption and consumption — because are these gut feelings my organs are having or feelings I am having at the expense of my gut — by ultimately finding the gut–brain space to be a space of decentralization, I am really saying that the visceralized body is not about biological determinism. How could this be possible? How could a physicality-reinforcing body be outside of such reductionism? But consider the following as a definition of biological determinism: "To be determined by biology is to surrender to limitations, to deny the possibilities of change."[18] "Surrender" is like "innate resistance." It is constituted in part by its generation through or in proximity to an able body. "Surrender" is only seen as such when what is being surrendered is a form of ideal, universalized ability. Able bodies are not supposed to have limits; to acknowledge and surrender to limitations is inherently to acknowledge a lack of an able body. Even in theory, this lack should be avoided.

The visceralized body has its limitations.

---

18 Lynda Birke, *Feminism and the Biological Body* (New Brunswick, NJ: Rutgers University Press, 2000), 1.

What, actually, is wrong with acknowledging these limitations? I understand that when the idea of "surrender to limitations" is applied to gendered bodies, when limitations become identity constituting, such limitations or just the idea of them, or when the idea of them is taken as fact, become hugely problematic. But, within a sick visceralized body, when I am reading that sentence I am being asked to think about the limits of my body only in terms of surrender, including a surrender to the fact that this sentence, like so many others, is written in a way that "limitations" is implicitly taken to mean limitations as only applying to a gendered body; an able body, limitless as it is, is never mentioned. The surrender becomes one of a surrender to the limitations of ableism.

The limitations of the visceralized body are "actual" as much as theoretical. Limitations are physical. Like, taking care of baby while receiving chemotherapy must be shaped by limitations like exhaustion or nausea. Like, how I run, but only within a certain radius of my home in case I need to run home. Like, how often I don't go out. Like, how difficult it is to hold a job. What is really the problem with surrendering to these limitations? What is the problem with surrendering to the difficulties of caring for a newborn while receiving chemo if it means you may receive more support from family or friends? What is the problem with not wanting to find a word other than surrender if this is what feels accurate? Is "acceptance" any better? What is the problem with wanting a sentence about a surrender to limitations in which "limitations" is not inherently negative, surrender feels accurate and realistic, unapologetically physical? And following such a sentence, a moment where surrender, like a coworker's surrender, becomes visceral and the limitations of other's bodies become felt as and in one's own?

"To be determined by biology" can also mean several different things to a visceralized body, most of which depend on what "biology" is taken to mean. If "biology" means the physical body, and particularly the way that the body, the inside of it, is thought of as a separate, purely biological sphere ("purely" separate from the mind) and the way this biological body becomes full of hidden-from-view processes then, yes, the visceralized body is determined by biology. If biology is taken to include medical science and human biology then, yes, the visceralized body is determined by biology. Because if I didn't follow my doctor's advice, if I didn't have advice from doctors with decades of pancreas-specific training, there would only be a body to bury, not a body to be determined. On the other hand, if biology is taken to mean something purely scientific, as if science was something that just happened, as if biology wasn't a thing that people do, then the visceralized body is not determined by biology. Because what biology can mean, what it actually must mean, etymologically, is not at all something that can just be discovered: it is a "study of." Studying, like observation, like thinking, like rumination. The visceralized body is an ongoing study.

I understand the problematic nature of biological determinism, the way that biology is and has been used to make universalizing claims about bodies applied particularly to Other(ed) bodies and the way that disciplines emerging from biology, like medicine and genetics, are used to reinforce norms of Otherness and inferiority. I understand the physical effects this kind of "biology" has on bodies and I am not arguing that a continued interrogation of this form of biological determinism within theory is irrelevant. But the way this form of biological determinism is written into theory such that it is taken as applicable to only racial, gendered, or queer others is itself a determining gesture. Even "disability studies," with its focus on social construction, tends to downplay or ignore or deny the biology within and behind disabled bodies. Which is to say: the rhetoric of anti-biological determinism gets rid of biological bodies along with biology. It is as if all of this theoretical work takes biology to be a definitive answer.

Because of biology, medicine creates and enforces bodily norms. Because of biology, people of color have been subject to centuries of oppression, fueled by fields like eugenics or phrenology. Because of biology, hormonal and neurological "causes" for LGBTQ people are being sought, because with that kind (any kind) of difference, there must be a locatable source. For a visceralized body, biology is never an answer but a question. The visceralized body is (in) an ongoing study. Is my gut sad because of biology? Does shit happen because of biology? Will biology make me feel better?

Probably not, but neither will structuralism nor social construction.

When I read sentences with words like determined and surrender and limitations, when these words could be about my body but never are, I feel like I'm in a space, like a hole, like a tunnel, that's empty. If a fear of biological determinism becomes formulated through an intense theoretical anti-biological determinism, anti-biology, what it has created is exactly this hole: the hole of theoretical determinism. A hole that envelops, tunnels fully around, the visceralized body.

I can understand why biology might be scary, in addition to fueling gender-, race-, or sex-based discrimination. Am I going to get sick suddenly (again) because of biology? Will I die earlier than I would have (if I didn't get sick) because of biology? How much shit happens because of biology? Is my gut sad because of biology? How much biology can a body take?

Does biology really happen in this way, though? Or is it more like: TBD by biology. More like: it's up in the air and biology is the question. More like: there are definitely social aspects of being sick that exacerbate it, but in no way did I get sick because of social or external factors alone. Even in cases with clear external causes, a body is just responding, biologically, however it can.

One person who did know how it feels was Oliver Sacks. Writing about a loss of sensation in his leg following an accidental fall and a surgery, he realized that this loss was something many of his patients had similarly experienced: "[E]very single one of them has this fear — known it and been unable to share it." The fear is one of loss and specifically a loss of "the sense of part of their body."[19] Oliver Sacks knew how much being unable to know comes to constitute what it feels like.

In writing further about this experience, Sacks pointed to a key part of such a visceral loss. On his own leg he says that "not only was I unable to perceive the leg, I was in some sense unable to remember it." He uses the term "amnesia."[20] The temporal relationship such an amnesia describes is one of "having/had." Like, having/had cancer. Or, for the visceralized body, having/had a sense of a body where nothing was like a hole, like a tunnel, both remembers this sense and feels an amnesiac lack of memory about what exactly this felt like. If you don't know how something feels, now, how can you remember what it felt like when, before, it felt like nothing? Or, the

19 Oliver Sacks, "The Leg," *London Review of Books* 4.11, June 17, 1982, https://www.lrb.co.uk/v04/n11/oliver-sacks/the-leg.
20 Sacks, "The Leg."

visceralized body having/had the loss of "the sense of part of their body," now feels everything keenly because in the face of a lack of information every single small piece comes to feel important.

Having/had becomes a temporal relationship useful to clarifying the way I am using the term "loss." Because having/had is a time frame that includes the possibility of ongoing conditions, the experience and memory of finished past conditions, and imperfect past conditions. A loss of sensation is not the same as an absence of sensation. Having/had does not create only a (permanent) surrender and limitations.

Oliver Sacks, in this same article, also provided the best term for condensing what I mean when I say that the gut is a hole, like a tunnel, but not empty: "negative phantom." He uses "negative phantom" to describe the way that his leg felt like a phantom limb yet paradoxically was still very much present and attached to his body. The gut is a negative phantom. The gut is a negative phantom and the power of unknowingness it can generate is such that maybe I knew (somewhere — felt) even more than I realized when I said "ghostbody."

Absent-Minded

Another term I didn't have yet, when I did have ghostbody, was theoretical determinism. Theoretical determinism: the way that critical theory shapes experiences of bodies. The way that critical theory writes bodies, provides information about bodies, in such a way as to directly affect the experience of readers' bodies. The way that, because of anti-biological determinism, because of the way this demanded that scholars get rid of biology, with or without deciding whether biology was "purely" scientific or a thing people do or a body, as in physical matter, means that the only body in critical theory now is The Body. The Body is a product of theoretical determinism. The Body is capitalized because it is more like a slogan or a brand name than a body; because it is just a cipher, because it, as a hollow figure, can hold whatever things, whatever things people do, in it.

Gut Reaction

I know I'm not the first to say this, that the body functions as a cipher within critical theory. See James Porter: "The mere concept of the body shields theory from its objects; it prevents us from confronting the body in any other way than as a fascination."[21] I know that theories of bodies as entirely social constructions are not without their discontents. But I also know that as much as there may be cries about "The Absent Body," it is still necessary to say (over and over) that it is the sick body that is made especially absent.

It is as if no one will admit to sickness.

Absent-Minded

Theoretical determinism is why I have been saying, here, repeatedly, that there is no information. Because in the same way that biology can be taken to mean the physical body and medicine and the study of both, by information I mean both medical information (like a diagnosis, like what does "damage" mean? Like what does "permanent" mean?), phenomenological information from first- or secondhand sources (like will my coworker tell me how it feels?) and theoretical information (like an analysis of first- or secondhand accounts of the phenomenology of illness, or like *Being Sick and Time,* or like *Illness Not As Metaphor*). Theoretical information is a structure that acts as a full realization of the term "framework:" because it provides a frame through which to see (you, your body, your experiences), a support onto which other information or experiences can be put, and it involves a certain amount of work, both the work of seeing as well as the work of building up and experiencing.

When I say that I want *Being Sick and Time* or *Illness Not As Metaphor,* I don't mean to say that I want a readymade framework or one that allows me to not put in any work. I mean: how different my experience of my body (and my time, and my relationships, and my future) would have been if I had been able to read *Being Sick and Time* years ago, if I had known (more, differently), about how

21 James Porter, "[The Body in Theory]," *Public Culture* 11.3 (1990): 440–42; 441.

it could feel. It could have been a framework that could have helped to fill in, in small parts, at least, other medical or phenomenological information that was also (still) missing.

Gut Reaction

At the same time, theory isn't everything. Maybe I would never have felt I needed *Being Sick and Time* if I had only been a little sick or if it didn't last. I didn't, actually, at first, want *Being Sick and Time*. I was content to just read *Being and Time*. Theoretical determinism tunnels slowly. Because it took years of reading, took years of sentences about "surrender" and "limitations" as well as sentences about "impairment" and "disability studies" to realize that none of these sentences described my body. To realize that I in no way have A Body.

Absent-Minded

It took longer for me to see how this failure to describe, to just leave my body out of it, was not a neutral act of exclusion. As if you just didn't have room in your word count. It was and is an act of exclusion predicated on exactly the same kind of reductionism involved in biological determinism. Because theoretical determinism reduces bodies to The Body, reduces experiences of yourself as/in a body to you as A Body: instead of the "you are your body" of biological determinism, theoretical determinism means that you are what is made of you. You are what is seen of you. You are what cultural factors determine you to be. In a perfect neoliberal shift, you are what you make of yourself.

Theoretical determinism is a hole, like a tunnel, around the body, that mirrors the hole of the gut. Theoretical determinism is a hole because The Body is constituted by cultural factors, because The Body is (only) what is seen, and so the hole is like a trap, one covered by camouflaging ground. Theoretical determinism reduces the body only to its surface. And uses this surface, spreads it, to cover the depth of the hole left in its reductionist wake. Theoretical determinism renders the inside of the body empty.

Gut Reaction

Maybe I didn't want *Being Sick and Time* at first because critical theory, as strong a framework as it may be, doesn't exactly make being sick better.

Absent-Minded

The exclusion of the body through theoretical determinism, while in and of itself is not neutral, has, in some ways, passed neutrally through decades of scholarship. That is, both the hole of The Body and the exclusion of other bodies have both passed neutrally, as in with little notice, through those decades. Which is something I've been trying to say, more or less successfully, for some time now. Something I've tried to say in multiple ways, like when I said "compulsory able bodiedness."[22] It's not that this was wrong, just somewhat incomplete. Compulsory able bodiedness has also been noted before, by others, as a way to name the ways in which space, cultural and physical, is shaped for and by able bodies. But theoretical space is not without its shaping factors either. It seems like philosophical lineage is something that should be easy to trace, to locate references and vocabulary and the movement of ideas, cohesively; it's easy to see this as a space more or less shaped freely. That is, more or less unshaped by unacknowledged ideologies.

But see, even now, when I am trying to just say the thing I've been trying to say, it's like I have to, like I can only, tell you through this kind of grounding lineage. Like this lineage is the only thing capable of grounding and validating ideas.

The thing about this lineage, though, and the space it creates, is a feature of its foundation: the entire history of Western metaphysics and philosophy is based on an able body.

Gut Reaction

It's funny, because in a lot of ways, for years, I have been angrier about this fact than I have been about being sick. It's funny, because

---

22 Maia Dolphin-Krute, *Ghostbodies: Towards a New Theory of Invalidism* (Bristol, UK: Intellect, 2017), 69.

this is easier to be angry about than being sick. It's funny, because this is also something that it feels easier to do something about.

Absent-Minded

In her book *Ongoingness,* Sarah Manguso writes about her practice of diary keeping, which spanned decades. She adds to these documents every day, sometimes more. She describes this intensely daily process as "more than daily."

"More than daily" is how I would describe the able body that is the basis of all metaphysics, of phenomenology, of The Body. This more-than-dailyness is what makes compulsory able bodiedness seem incomplete. Because that concept is taken from the idea of compulsory heterosexuality, which itself depends on the idea that heterosexuality is positioned as "wholly natural."[23] What doesn't fit about this, here, is that able bodiedness is more than natural. The able body is the thing that makes (human) nature possible, the able body is the thing that is more natural than anything else. Compulsory able bodiedness names a condition of invisibility. But the way that the able body is the basis of The Body, the way that this foundational fact has been able to pass neutrally through so much work, is more than invisible. It is a force that I have also elsewhere called a prototype; but the able body, again, is more like the prototype on which all others are based. It shapes The Body because it is (only, always, right?) the body. It shapes The Body, and it is the body, and this seems so neutral because doesn't "human," doesn't the body, only ever mean one that is definitively alive, one that isn't sick, one whose wholeness is never threatened, one whose mind is and can remain superior, one whose inside is never distracting, one that isn't stuck in its hole of a gut; a body that is these qualities is never The Body. The Body, in the way it writes the body, in the way it excludes these possibilities, deploys the very idea of the body in an almost absent-minded way. More than daily. More than invisible. More than taken for granted. It's like no one will admit to sickness.

---

23 Robert McRuer, *Crip Theory: Cultural Signs of Queerness and Disability* (New York: New York University Press, 2006), 151.

Gut Reaction

Is biology really so scary?

Absent-Minded

Sickness is something that needs to be admitted. Sickness takes up space. Sickness pushes other things aside; sickness distorts the boundaries of The Body. Sickness is a thing that must have room made for it. Sickness is a thing that pushes aside the more-than-invisibleness of The Body.

No one will admit to sickness because, in a body where the mind is and can remain superior, where embodiment is something that can be studied in way closely bordering on "detached," there is no room for threats from things, from biology, that theoretical determinism has judged inferior.

The visceralized body, with its holes, like tunnels, but not empty, has room for sickness.

Theoretical determinism has no room for sickness. Theoretical determinism drives theory to tunnel fully around sick bodies, because sickness is too large an obstacle; sickness cannot be reduced. The able body, the way that the able body is a prototype before all other prototypes, is the ultimate reduction. It is the easiest reduction (so clean! so whole! so able!) and therefore the easiest starting point. It is the easiest starting point on which to pile on all those cultural factors. It is the easiest starting point, the most common of common denominators, because it ultimately erases the source of the greatest variation and difference and, simultaneously, same-nesses, among people; it reduces all of this to The Body. It eliminates the problems of bodies. It, more than invisibly, eliminates any notice of this until, suddenly, The Body is no longer possible, until it is no longer possible to imagine yourself in A Body while reading about Bodies; until it becomes clear that the able body is not your prototype. And then where is *Being Sick and Time*?

Absent-Minded (Again, Differently)

Or: sick is not a quality. Sick is not an aspect or feature or trait. Sick cannot be reduced through theoretical determinism because sick is a sheer physical fact. Sick is always already in its simplest, essential, form. Theoretical determinism cannot reduce it and so it just tunnels fully around it; by completely excluding sick, by making its absence more than invisible, theoretical determinism neutralizes sick; it makes the absence of sickness (within theory) seem neutral.

Saying "sick" is in its simplest and most essential form is not the same as saying that being sick lacks complexity. If theoretical determinism creates a tunnel, the visceralized body provides a form capable of moving through such a tunnel, provides a way of giving complexity to sickness, to being sick, while never ignoring (because how do you not feel something in your own body, including the absence of sensation) physical fact (which is a fact that announces itself physically, which is why it can't be ignored, because how do you ignore urgency in your own body).

I'll admit to sickness.

Just because I asked for *Being Sick and Time* doesn't mean that I haven't been able to find anything else. It's just a matter of application. Like this, another consideration of the space of "able body," from Foucault in "Madness, the Absence of Work:" "It will not be said that we were at a distance from madness, but within distance of it."[24] It cannot be said that we ("we," able bodies) are at a distance from sickness but always constituted in part by being within a distance of it.

He goes on in that essay to write that, in relation to said distances, there exists "this desire to establish the limit yet at once to compensate for it through the framework of unitary meaning."[25] The able body is the limit. It sets the limits of The Body. To compensate for this limit, sickness (people who are sick) becomes the object ground down to the anchoring (as in holding in place, deeply, as in suctioning, as in this is not comfortable or comforting, as in weighing down) surface of "able body." The unification of the able body with its limits is made in the idea (the framework) that sickness is a thing that happens (not that just *is*), that sickness is socially constructed (that it happens, somewhere else, somewhere at a distance to the

24 Michel Foucault, "Madness, the Absence of Work," trans. Peter Stastny and Deniz Sengel, *Critical Inquiry* 21.2 (1995): 290–98; 292.

25 Foucault, "Madness, the Absence of Work," 293.

able body). That sickness is a thing that happens, that it is not an inherent (or natural) flaw in the surface of the able body.

The limit of the able body is also its limited capacity to make itself felt (in all senses).

Gut Reaction

Writing about her experiences caring for her son, who has neurological impairments, Julia Kristeva refers to the urgency and utopian nature of negotiating for disability rights and the day-to-day negotiations of being sick.[26] This urgency can be blinding. This urgency has been a main difficulty in my trying to name the able body and The Body here, the source of so much messiness. This urgency is my limit, though this is really just the product of moving urgently on slippery surfaces; skidding.

Absent-Minded

Theoretical determinism is the compensation for the limits of the able body. Sickness is the only limit that matters. Sickness must be admitted but will, can, never truly be. To compensate, theoretical determinism admits so much else; it admits socially constructed bodies and marginalized identities and systemic oppression enacted through (seemingly) bodiless modes of corporate, governmental, and institutional neglect.

But it cannot admit, cannot reduce to the level of human action, sickness; it cannot admit that sickness is a thing that *is*.

This has always been about this limit. Not that that has always been recognizable. Not that there have always been the words to name this.

Gut Reaction

It took my sad gut, realizing its sadness, feeling it, not being able to feel it, to come to these words. This seems like the opposite of the popular theoretical rhetoric surrounding pain, the idea that pain is

26 Julia Kristeva, "A Tragedy and A Dream: Disability Revisited," *Irish Theological Quarterly* 78.3 (2013): 219–30.

resistant to language, that it dissolves words. So what does it mean for a sad gut, for a visceral experience, to have actually provided the words "the able body is the basis of Western metaphysics and philosophy"? What does it mean that one (but not singular) personal experience of the limit of perception made clear a much larger limit, a lack of information? It means that maybe the body, maybe pain or sickness, is nowhere near as language-resistant as has been thought. It means that experiencing within a visceralized body opens new areas of knowledge. Because even learning of a lack of information itself generates understanding. Because when there is not enough information about my body, about my sick body, within my body itself, why is it that there is nowhere else to look for and find such information? Why are there no words? Because it is not pain that takes away words; it just makes clear their need. It is not pain that takes away words; it is the able body. The able body is the lack.

I don't want a medical narrative, I want a theoretical narrative.

Even recognizing this grinding, slipping, reducing, reductive, force at the heart of critical theory, why does theory remain desirable? Even before that question, the answer to which is about the work that theory does, it could be asked whether the able body is even a problem for theory at all. Who cares? Who is theory for? (Ask that of my sad gut, asshole.) Why does theory remain desirable even if, as it is now, it is really only for people in an able body (or who want one, or who can think about having one), people who can believe in The Body?

Because I don't want a medical narrative, I want a theoretical narrative. Because medical narratives are always already filled in but theoretical narratives are open space, space that can open around. Because medical narratives are inescapable. Which I say even though I hate the word "inescapable" but it's also true; theoretical narratives are open to (for) escape. Theoretical narratives are about possibilities. I don't want a medical narrative not because I'm opposed to progress or getting better but because I would rather (given the odds, given the day-to-day work involved in a medical sense of better) think about what else "better" can mean. Because theory is easier than being sick. Because being sick makes theory (more) possible, makes theory a possibility. Because being sick and theory both turn everything into possibilities.

Because I have the right to a theoretical narrative.

Because when you are sick and reading and/or producing theory, when everything is a possibility, narratives are never linear. A theoretical narrative both matches the time of a visceralized body and provides a way out of it. Like, is my gut sad because of theory? Do I not know what my gut is because of theory? How can I think about this unknown? How much theory can a body take? How much non-linearity can a body take? How many escapes can a body be provided? If it's better that pain becomes language-generating instead of language-resistant, how many words must be found to "make it worthwhile?" How much, of what, is "worthwhile"? Worthwhile "in theory" or "in life?"

In theory, and in the lineage that I am thinking of here, backwards from disability studies to queer studies to feminist critical theory to Simone de Beauvoir to Lacan and Freud, is one based on an able body whose main attribute (or defining characteristic) is sexuality. That is, the person's sexuality, because the main work of feminist critical thought was to separate the biological body from the mind, the mind that produces (enacts) "the female" on/through/upon the body. It is this enactment that ultimately produces The Body. It is this enactment and performativity of such a foundational aspect of identity that makes it seem so obvious that the rest of identity is an enactment as well. This follows through feminist critical theory to queer studies to critical race theory, to examinations of the socially, linguistically, constructed experiences of queerness or race. Which, in turn, continues in examinations of all other aspects of identity, including being disabled.

Enactment is what makes invalids. How can you theorize an enactment of identity when it takes place in a body that itself is enacting both "alive" and "dead"? (Ignore the body.) How can you theorize an enactment of identity in a body that is never in one place long enough for anything to be enacted upon it? (Ignore the body.) How can you theorize an enactment of identity upon a body whose surface is meaningless, when confronted with the even more meaningful meaninglessness of its insides? How do you enact being dead, but still alive, now?

Because being dead cannot be enacted, being sick cannot be either. This is not such a stretch; being sick is not the same as being dead but nor is it ever really very different; it cannot be said that we were at a distance from being sick, but within distance of it. When being sick is seen as an identity, when disability studies theorizes itself into being, invalids are made. Because it is not enough to talk about sickness as a thing that happens or a thing people do. Because how does it feel? Because having words is not enough without also having information.

The thing about all of this theory, about feminist and queer and disability studies, is that this is not just about a lineage of erasure and no words and non-identity. This is not just about lineage, as if lineage were just a thing that happened, a history. This is not just about lineage because this is also how I was taught. I was taught that this is what critical theory is. I was taught that this is what is included within critical theory. I was taught this lineage. I was given readings. I was not taught about being sick, although I have been sick for six years and could have a Masters by now. It is the lineage of critical theory that is enacted.

Gut Reaction

The ironic thing about a difference constituted by sickness or disability is that this is actually a difference based on the most same of samenesses. The real difference is not the sickness itself but an awareness, even if it's an awareness of the limits of perception. An awareness of the limits of information.

I also cannot unlearn what I was taught about critical theory and its lineage. It's a lineage taught and enacted by people who can still think, comfortably, of The Body. What is taught through this Body is a paradigm in which the object of theory is identity, in which identity is constituted as a set series of differences from established norms, and that the most transgressive differences are those concerning sexuality and gender. "Everyone shifted over from production to perversion."[27] Coming out of Freud and Lacan, critical theory is based on The Body as (only ever) the sexualized body.

The visceralized body is not the sexualized body.

27 Terry Eagleton, "It is not quite true that I have a body and not quite true that I am one either," *London Review of Books* 15.10, July 22, 1993, http://www.lrb.co.uk/v15/n10/terry-eagleton/it-is-not-quite-true-that-i-have-a-body-and-not-quite-true-that-i-am-one-either.

I cannot unlearn what I was taught about differences and norms, but, within such a system, how can you think about a difference predicated on the most normal norm? Being alive, but dying, is the most basic, unavoidable, norm. Sickness is no different.

When I said that I have a right to a theoretical narrative, what I meant was that I have the right to theory centered not on the sexualized body but on the visceralized body. The visceralized body can serve not only as a way to talk about visceral bodily experiences, it can also be a model for theory; it can be a new paradigm. And, indeed, it would have to be a new paradigm, because how can you write sickness within a theoretical paradigm where sickness cannot be admitted? Only ever partially.

Was disability studies supposed to be the new paradigm? Was crip theory? A huge amount of the work of disability studies has been a "positioning [of] disability as a set of practices and associations that can be critiqued, contested and transformed."[28] But this work has been exactly the kind of enactment that writes out sick bodies, that is (a) "set," that's "practices," that's "associations," but what does this actually mean for living in a body every day? Disability studies has continually pushed aside these issues, pushed aside messiness, to focus on questions framed as (only) larger (more important) political issues. Because theory is easier than being sick. I would suggest that a theory whose object is the visceralized body is less about contestation or transformation and more in line with *Being Sick and Time*: an elucidation, a phenomenology, a filling in of gaps. Thinking in the gut–brain space. Being aware of the slippery surface of the able body. Being sick.

To not focus on contestation or critique, or at least what critique commonly means, doesn't mean that a theory of the visceralized body wouldn't be critical. To inhabit a hyperphysical, fully felt, body in a theoretical context where "bodies are ways of talking about human subjects without getting all sloppily humanist"[29] is inherently a critique of existing theoretical norms. Simply being aware of theoretical determinism is critical. Sloppiness can be critical. Shit is critical.

28 Alison Kafer, *Feminist, Queer, Crip* (Bloomington, IN: Indiana University Press, 2013), 9.
29 Eagleton, "It is not quite true."

Was disability studies supposed to be the new paradigm? What does it mean to find that this doesn't include sickness? It begs the question of defining sickness as something opposed to disability, an easy definition to fall into. But my issues with disability studies have less to do with how disability is commonly defined and more to do with how it is written as a "set of practices and associations," as something that almost always visibly marks a body, something that has more to do with wheelchairs and ramps than shit and guts. Something also generally written as a permanent state, probably something you were born with. Something that feels static, something that never includes or admits to being in pain every day, something that never makes you have to discuss diarrhea with your partner. And no, sickness is not always these (static) things. It is less aligned with the freaks paradigm of disability studies and more about ghosts and the walking dead and the undead; less about obvious monstrosity and more about figuring out what, exactly, is monstrous.

On the other hand, what does it really matter whether sickness and disability are mutually exclusive terms? At least within theory, because there are definite legal implications for how disability is defined, which I don't mean to ignore and to which we will return later. But, here, within theory, whether sickness can or should be considered a disability should be something of a nonissue. First and foremost because defining bodies, defining bodies by their conditions and practices and associations, will always end up at The Body. By focusing on disability as such, by relying on and reinforcing definitive differences between disability and people with disabilities and impairments, disability studies only winds up writing Another Body. Even (or especially) crip theory, which, in part, seeks to better integrate disability studies with queer theory, to be more inclusive, but must first define that which it includes. All of this defining is an attempt to avoid sloppiness. Or to avoid a confrontation.

Secondly, shifting away from a theory focused on defining categories of identities to one based on the visceralized body also means a shift in vocabulary. This is why it doesn't really matter, within theory, whether disability and sickness are the same or mutually exclusive; everything is visceral. The visceralized body is open to others to the extent that it is not really necessary to first define what to be inclusive of. The visceralized body needs a theory understanding of the fact that theory is easier than being sick; why close it off?

Was the category of being sick ever that much of a difference? At first, I thought that perhaps the lack of sickness within disability studies was because, historically, sickness really was that distinct, and so it would, now, be more accurate to say that sickness is no longer a difference. And I could see why this could be true, I could see how the huge rise of conditions like obesity and diabetes make it seem like suddenly everyone is sick; now that so many people are sick, it's like sickness is no longer a difference. But, on the other hand, people have always been sick. People have always been sick and historically even more people have been sick than are sick now and even more people have died, often at home, from sicknesses the majority of which are no longer fatal. This, actually, is the only real difference, now, that the majority of people no longer expect to get sick and die. Especially given that with so many diseases being made nonfatal, now, many more people will be walking around sick; alive, but maybe already a little dead. Sickness is both not the norm, now, even as it once was, and simultaneously, is still the most basic norm. If the able body is the most natural natural, sickness is the most normal difference. It invalidates itself.

Absent-Minded

I want to return to these legal implications of "disabled" now, specifically to think about obesity. Because it's not just that with the rise of obesity and diabetes there are suddenly millions (more) sick people. It is also the fact that with the declaration that obesity is a disability, there are suddenly millions (more) disabled people in the US. Further, the more or less concurrent passage of the Affordable Care Act included within its provisions ones that directly affect the protection of sick people; in a way, creating legal protections similar to those already in place for the protection of disability rights. For example, the fact that the law made it illegal for insurance companies to refuse to cover or raise charges for people with pre-existing conditions meant that millions of chronically ill people had their right to accessible health care protected.

But what do these legal rights have to do with theory? There is more than one lineage to theory. When looking at a history of disability studies, there is a remarkable concurrence of successful disability rights activism with an increase in the popularity of disability studies. Like how the passage of the ADA in 1990 happened during a period, from about 1990–1995, that saw a large amount of sociological scholarship about illness and disability produced. This production slowed to a halt in about 1995 — more or less the time that the release of protease inhibitors and their success in turning AIDS from a death sentence to a chronic illness (which itself is a kind of right) happened, meaning that there were now very many less sick people. It no longer seemed like a crisis, of health or attention. Now, between crip theory and disability studies, The Disabled are everywhere; this rise seems to have happened within the past 10–15 years, as debates about rights like the ACA raged. Debates, and media surrounding the debates, and scholarship done at the time, brings to mind Rosemarie Garland-Thompson's writing about freak shows and their relationship to disabled bodies: "The immense popularity of the shows between the Jacksonian and Progressive eras suggest that the onlookers needed to constantly reaffirm the difference between 'them' and 'us' at a time when immigration, emancipation of the slaves and female suffrage confounded previously reliable physical indices of status and privilege."[30] The immense popularity of disability studies between 2000 and 2015 suggests the need to constantly reaffirm the difference between "them" and "us" at a time that's included the passage of the ACA, the declaration that obesity is a disability and rising rates of autism, diabetes, and autoimmune diseases (for example): Who's disabled now?

I am not normally disabled.

The people who are disabled now are not depicted as freaks, but as the direct opposite, as incredibly mundane, unexceptional, because of the huge number of Americans affected. The people who are disabled now are not freaks but they are "the obesity epidemic," which, although not "freak," has the same effect. "The obesity epidemic" names millions of people, makes it seem like these sick bodies are everywhere, but, by naming these people as singular, renders them invisible. "The obesity epidemic" is everywhere and nowhere at once.

It can't possibly, really, be your problem.

30 McRuer, *Crip Theory,* 103.

"The obesity epidemic" is not at a distance from "disabled" but within distance of it. But any distance here is crucial because what would it mean for, suddenly, millions of people to now be disabled? Can you be disabled by an illness? Can you be disabled by an illness that seems to have such clear external causes, causes like food deserts and HFCS and a lack of educational and health resources? An illness that seems to be both physically present, in that it has clear physical effects, and remarkably disembodied. What will these bodies mean for other disabled bodies, bodies whose disabilities seem so physical, so definite, and solid? Sickness can't possibly be admitted. It can't possibly be your problem, because with an illness like obesity you can just avoid those behaviors that cause it. And then not get sick. And then maintain your distance. And then.

I am tempted to say: what does it matter what effects obesity will have on the larger category of disabled? It's not that I don't understand the fact of limited resources, the distribution or lack thereof of such resources, to all kinds of bodies. But, theoretically, linguistically, (empathetically,) why isn't there room for admitting these bodies? If your body is legally protected, why can't it be theoretically protected?

The bodilessness of obesity, the way it is seemingly constituted by only actions, not internal mechanisms, actually makes it a perfect test case for illustrating the possibilities of thinking through and around and with a visceral body. Because obese bodies are bodies that are experiencing the very physical effects of an illness that (they are being told) is a product of their behaviors, of their minds, of the minds and behaviors of those around them. Obese bodies are bodies existing within and experiencing (and exemplifying) the gut–brain space. Obese bodies can make this space apparent in ways that more invisibly ill bodies may not be able to (at first). Obese bodies are visceral bodies. Furthermore, the obesity epidemic has seen a huge rise in nutrition studies, in the evaluation of various diets, in the long-term tracking of various metabolic data. What these data show, and the metabolic data in particular, is concurrent rise of people who have health problems identical to those caused by obesity, despite their non-obese weight: the term is metabolically obese normal weight. Who is disabled now? How is sickness any different?

Gut Reaction

The visceral bodies of the obesity epidemic, and the inherent inseparability of mind and body when considering their illness, coupled
with historical concurrence of disability rights activism and disability rights studies, makes clear that now is the time for rights. Not
just further legal rights. And it's not disability studies that's needed,
now, not work that works on definitions, but theoretical rights that
collapse definitions and works towards more information. Theoretical rights that respond to the inseparability of mind and body
in a visceral body; that recognize that visceral bodies deserve legal
rights that attend to physical needs as much as they deserve theoretical rights that attend to the need for information. Rights in theory;
rights to a narrative in theory. Rights to *Being Sick and Time*. And
rights to *Illness Not As Metaphor* but also rights to seeing or doing
the rewriting and reapplying of existing theoretical narratives to visceral bodies. Like what if, for once, a discussion of Foucault's *Discipline and Punish* was about the different power dynamics within a
body, about varying cellular or organ level regulatory mechanisms
and what these mechanisms could show about larger political or
social systems? What if Kristeva's concept of the abject was taken
to include the things one's body finds abject within itself, like all
that shit or those food intolerances or a faulty autoimmunity?
What if différance/difference wasn't just about the linguistics of
terms, the play, but the way the negation inherent in them applies
to the non-difference of sickness? What if, to continue with Der-
rida, an idea of a specter could be used to think about a specter of
saturation (as related to rumination)? What if the author is actually
dead or dying? What if there was a body of text that was disjointed,
tongue-in-cheek, where the argument really didn't have a leg to
stand on; what if there were a sick body of text? What if, these questions answered, these theoretical rights fulfilled, then what? "What
should I be cured of? To find what condition, what life?"[31]

---

31 Roland Barthes, *Mourning Diary* (New York: Hill & Wang, 2010), 97.

Daily Survivor #2
(Living With, or An Afterword)

All of the time, I work.

I would like to have a nice life. I would like to have a nice life with many things in it. I imagine these things as being more or less easily separated from my life or the things in my body. I work at imagining as much as I work at pulling apart.

How do you live with something for a long time?

* * *

My doctor thinks I should run off and live my life. These are more or less his exact words: ride off on a horse, he tells me. Presumably because I am not quite like his other pancreatitis patients. I can still ride a horse, definitely. I have not (very) recently suffered a catastrophic illness. As he reminded me at our last appointment, I do still have a pancreas. I'm not facing an average 15-year post-diagnosis survival rate? Does he know something I don't? Or is the opposite true, does he think that this is, in fact, exactly what I'm facing and therefore should find those horses while I can? Either way, the attitude is the same: take advantage now, enjoy now, because there is (maybe) no next. Does it really matter why not? Regardless, all of the time I imagine the "maybe" becoming my present: I fall down the stairs carrying my laundry out. Someone knocks into me at work. Accidently, I eat something I shouldn't. And these are not truly, or only, scenarios within my imagination. Every day I do these things or work to avoid them. See, once, during a conversation after a series of events involving months of negotiation with my insurance company, a definitive diagnosis of chronic pancreatitis, a colonoscopy the day before Thanksgiving, and the removal of a precancerous intestinal growth I was told they would "never find in a 22-year-old," my mother said I would have to be diligent. The word got stuck in my head. I knew she was right, but also surprised by this word choice: why not careful, or patient? Diligence is the opposite of riding off. Both are living.

In imagining, mostly imagining becoming again very sick, I am not extravagant. The scenarios I imagine are intensely mundane, unavoidably so. A month ago, there was suddenly a sharp pain. I knew this pain. And I thought: maybe now is the next time. And so I went to the hospital and in the waiting room, during the first few minutes before I could do nothing but sit, change position minutely, and begin to cry, I wrote: "Now that it has come again, it is and is not like I imagined or remembered." In the waiting room I read *El Mundo*. My horoscope says that I will soon visit a special place. Later, I listen to a man getting an electrocardiogram five feet away from me in a hallway. I think, today I have.

It is not that either my doctor or my mother were right or wrong about diligence or running off. Living with is both of these, also neither of them, or is the desire and necessity of both, alternately and unavoidably continuously.

* * *

I start to read books about aging. That is almost like living with something for a long time, right? Or at least is just something that happens for a long time. Besides, I remain attached to a few age-related fantasies and figures. Middle age. Specifically, middle-aged men. How, statistically, I am one: I have the pancreatitis of middle-aged men, the precancerous intestinal growth of middle-aged men. The treatment plans and procedures determined because of these statistics on the bodies of the other middle-aged men. Even knowing the growths and organ damage involved, being middle-aged remains a fantasy. An odd one, maybe. Who wants to be 50? It seems like almost no one; I can't wait. In one sense, anyway, in that that will mean I have lived for another 25 years. At the same time, as I said, chronic pancreatitis has a 15-year post-diagnosis survival rate, though with diagnosis happening, on average, at 43. I would like to be nicely middle-aged.

I imagine myself reading this when I am very old. Or very sick. I will, I know, have gotten many things wrong, and I wonder what I will then find embarrassing. It won't really matter. This is not *Letters to a Young Poet,* it's *Letters to a Sick Young Poet.* It will turn out differently.

The funny thing about prognostic information for a disease you have but that may or may not apply to you (or, at least, may be 25 years out of sync with you) is how warped the idea of "old age" and the speed of "aging" become. You read: diabetes happens most often after about 20 years of illness. (I thought there would only be fifteen?) This seems like a long time. It seems like I'll be old then. But, then, I realize how I've already been sick for almost 6 years. It will both go very quickly and always seem like the longest time, a seemingly impossible temporal dichotomy: chronic. Intractable.

About those middle-aged men: the majority of them have alcohol-induced pancreatitis that has damaged the overall structure of the organ and, for this reason, is easy to visualize using existing imaging technologies like MRI and ultrasound. Young women, it is now increasingly being found, are more likely to have a kind of pancreatitis not specific to alcoholism, in which the majority of organ damage is to the small, internal network of ducts: small duct pancreatitis. As there does not yet exist imaging technology sensitive enough to show this damage, its possible severity, all existing treatment plans are based on the large duct pancreatitis of middle-aged men. Hence they become an inescapable fantasy and (imposed) reality. They make my body more and more like theirs. For instance, I take so many NSAIDs (non-steroidal anti-inflammatories) that I become convinced, having done some research, that these NSAIDs have caused me to stop ovulating.[1] And I am so surprised how neither my middle-aged male doctor nor my 75-year-old male doctor mentioned this possible side effect (albeit presumably rare, or rarely

---

1   See M. Akil, R.S. Amos, and P. Stewart, "Infertility may sometimes be associated with NSAID consumption," *Rheumatolgy* 35.1 (1996): 76–78, doi: 10.1093/rheumatology/35.1.76, and S. Stone et. al., "Non-Steroidal Anti-Inflammatory Drugs and Reversible Infertility," *Drug Safety* 25.8 (2002): 545–51.

noticed; one assumes the majority of women taking this many NSAIDs are over the age of 40 or 50 and would perhaps not notice this effect). They treat me in their image.

Sometimes, I remember how I used to get these stitches in my side as kid, while running or being out of breath. They were just stitches. I'm sure. But this pain in my side that I have now is the only side pain I can remember or imagine, and it creeps not only forwards but backwards. What if it has been longer than 5 years? At what point do you start counting? What if it's genetic? I remember, also, one of the first things I ever wrote about being sick: what is ill in chronic illness is time.

There's a term for this, one used commonly in writing and theory about chronic illness: living in prognosis. At its core, living in prognosis is about experiencing a continuous temporal flux, brought on, perhaps, by a feeling that it is "as if there were a right to a certain lifespan," and you are or are not really being granted this right. Furthermore, "prognostic time constantly anticipates a future."[2] Which is, in short, exactly what a prognosis is: an estimate, based on the current severity, expected progression, experience of bodies like yours, of how much of a future there will be for you. In this way, a prognosis is entirely and only about a measure of time. A prognosis is less good at predicting how this time will feel. "Living in prognosis" is therefore a useful term, and description (as elucidated by writers like Sarah Lochlann Jain and Jasbir Puar), for describing how it feels to have a prognosis, what its progression, its estimates, feel like.

What if, though, you do not have a prognosis, it is difficult to estimate, you do not exactly know when you first got sick (and therefore where you should be counting from) or all estimates are based on bodies yours may be more and more like but remain distinct enough from to not, fully, be applicable?

What if you are living not in prognosis, but in mortality rates?

* * *

Say it is a rather deadly disease. Like, maybe there is a 25% mortality rate during certain acute episodes, that this increases with each

2   Sarah Lochlann Jain, "Living in Prognosis: Toward an Elegiac Politics," *Representations* 98.1 (2007): 77–92; 81.

reoccurrence. Such a state, coupled with an inability to accurately predict episodes such as this, and the inapplicability of existing prognosis, would make "living in prognosis" not useful. This, instead, is "living in mortality rates," which can be used to describe at least one aspect of *living with*. After all, when statistics about the probability of survivorship are not applicable, it makes sense for these statistics to morph, in a way that necessitates a reliance, instead, on the likelihood of death. A different kind of anticipation, maybe. And what, exactly, is there to anticipate in living in mortality rates? It is not the constant anticipation of the future as in prognosis. It's not that there is no future, either. It's that you're already living (in) an impossible future. Living in the "could have died." Living in the known premalignant. Living in mortality rates and therefore living not among the survived, alive, bodies of prognostic information but among those excluded from prognosis: dead bodies and the feeling of this mass. In mass, at least there is a lot to live with.

By "impossible future" I mean exactly the future of the "could have died." Or would have. And how much *time,* in a historical sense, can create this distinction: formal guidelines for the diagnosis and treatment of acute pancreatitis (with the 25% mortality rate) were not developed and put out by organized medical groups until 1995. I was born in 1993. (The joke: they saw me coming!)

By "impossible future," I am drawing on Michael Ralph's notion of "surplus time," the idea, and feeling, of "a moment they should not have been able to experience based on the perceived itinerary."[3] Living in the "should not have been."

Or, perhaps most viscerally: living in the "been spreading."

Writing in "Living in Prognosis: Towards an Elegiac Politics," Lochlann Jain describes a woman whose "cancer had spread (had, in fact, been spreading during the interim of hope, of 'survivorship')."[4] And what does the "progressive" in "progressive chronic illness" mean if not always already *been spreading*? Living in the been spreading feels the most solid of these phrases to me, the one with the most mass. The one, really, with always more and more mass.

---

3   Michael Ralph, "Flirt[ing] With Death But 'Still Alive': The Sexual Dimensions of Surplus Time in Hip Hop Fantasy," *Cultural Dynamics* 18.1 (2006): 61–88; 79.

4   Jain, "Living in Prognosis," 77.

* * *

I know, this must sound hopeless. The attraction of "prognosis" is how it always holds open a future in which you live, disease-free. "Mortality rates" does not (or at least not in the same way) promise this but it does promise a known, knowable end; in this way, one altogether more easily imagined and dependable than a future of being disease-free. How easy is it, really, to imagine "25% survival rate in 5 years"? Yet having been very sick, before, it is easy to imagine becoming very sick again. Even if I am not always entirely right in my imagining. Furthermore, what kind of prognosis can there even be in a chronic illness? One that somehow disavows the very meaning of "chronic"? Is it not more hopeless to remain attached to a prognostic fantasy that ignores the reality, the mass, of what is progressive, of what has been spreading? The thing about chronic illness is that you are only a survivor (of a kind) up until the point at which you die: why not start there? "So thou shall feed on Death that feeds on men,/And Death, once dead, there's no more dying then."[5] Why not start with the middle age I get to be, now? With the old married couple, with the sadness, even, this can hold now? When hope remains a risk perhaps hope in "living in mortality rates" is exactly the persistence of these figures and images, how they persist despite being refigured temporally and the risk this presents, the risk of actually being (like) middle-aged at 23.[6] When hope is a risk, is it riskier to have a life sentence or a death sentence? If a prognosis, a poor one, is a death sentence, shouldn't an illness you have for a long time be a life sentence?

Maybe diligence itself is a form of hope: diligence towards hope, diligence in living with the feeling, the likelihood, of your death. Its mass. Also, hope in and as homeostasis: a biological hope in the form of a body practicing an intrinsic kind of diligence, one unique to matter. To mass.

I'll take it day by day.

5   William Shakespeare, "Sonnet 146," *Poets.org,* https://www.poets.org/poetsorg/poem/poor-soul-centre-my-sinful-earth-sonnet-146.
6   Jasbir K. Puar, "Prognosis Time: Towards a Geopolitics of Affect, Debility and Capacity," *Women & Performance: a journal of feminist theory* 19.2 (2009): 161–72; 163.

* * *

How does right now become right now? How do you get to a place where you're thinking about living, how to live, with something for a long time? The point at which you realize "a long time." How do you get to a place where you're thinking about living with something for a long time while also already doing the living? In a way, living in mortality rates (or in prognosis) papers over the reality of this boredom, how now just creeps up on you; mortality rates, while true, sounds also too melodramatic. It's not dramatic. It's just the slow, maybe over years, closing off of other possibilities until, of course, it's only this: and you will be living with this for a long time. It is that simple.

In becoming encroaching, now is enacted over many smaller moments. I'll take it day by day, because I have to. How will I get home today? What will I take to eat? And on and on. I plan to plan.

"The problems with which ill people struggle are often existential; their solutions are organizational."[7]

Slowly, more and more decisions. More constant awareness of needs. How do you sustain decision-making and diligent, boring planning for years? The feeling of always needing something is not a comfortable one. Perhaps because of this, I'm not always sure if it makes it harder or easier that I haven't been sick since I was born: I remember what it's like to not need.

There is, though, incentive for maintaining these daily plans: "[F]or nowadays, I feel like plans are all that stand between me and the end of my life."[8] Throughout *The Light of the World*, written after the death of her husband, Elizabeth Alexander talks a lot about edges; what she grasps onto, lingers on. This makes sense in the face of such enormous and specific loss. Every day, though, is a much less specific kind of loss, also because so much remains. I do not want to continue grasping.

Instead, I'll take it day by day.

7   Kathy Charmaz, *Good Days, Bad Days: The Self and Chronic Illness in Time* (New Brunswick, NJ: Rutgers University Press, 1993), 138.
8   Elizabeth Alexander, *The Light of the World: A Memoir* (New York City: Grand Central Publishing, 2015), 195.

* * *

The pain makes that difficult sometimes. And more so now, when I seem to have a problem with friction. Not only do I not want to continue grasping, I have also completely lost the ability to push, to push through the pain and exhaustion. I simply stop. I stop so much more frequently now than I used to. That, the ability to keep going, I do not quite remember or understand it now. What exactly was I relying on? And I think a lot about why this is, how many ways I can explain it: the medication side effects, the malnutrition. These are believable explanations, but not entirely true. Really, I think this is just the feeling of being an entire year sicker. That is the only true difference between this year and last year. A year of living in the been spreading.

Despite being occasionally haunted by the feeling or knowledge (on some level, physically) that this is the best it is going to be, probably for a long time, there is also an odd relief in simply acknowledging the feeling of this progression. I try to convince myself I am just relaxing, not fighting, not just giving up.

The pain makes it hard sometimes. I've written so much about it before, described it in so many ways, I'm not sure what else there is to say. Except for how it's always changing, also always the same, and always surprising, so that even in describing it over and over again, I am always a little right and a little wrong. Every time, it is like I am trying to tell myself as much as you. As if only in finally describing it accurately will it get better. It becomes endlessly fascinating in this way, "fascinating" in a tactile sense, like turning something over again and again, some things becoming worn away. I try out sentences and phrases. I try to explain it to myself: chronic inflammation leads to scar tissue; acute inflammation causes higher and higher levels of enzyme production, digestive enzymes that can't tell the difference between the matter of the pancreas and the matter of food, how you digest yourself; how of course it has begun to hurt when I lift my right arm, everything being connected, encroaching, right?; how anti-inflammatories act chemically, how opiates attach to receptors in your brain stem; so much hard science, so many kinds of cells, just cells, as if, over and over, the hardness of this science can block out, through sheer force, how much these words are responsible for, how much I cannot always stand it.

So, I take it day by day.

* * *

The ironic thing about living with, at least sometimes, is how it also feels like my body is made of nothing. How there is nothing inside to be metabolized, to produce; the feeling of running on empty, but total. I am also living with (this feeling of) nothing.

I am not living with very well because of this nothing. It makes it difficult to do things like hold a job, or work at one enough days out of the week to make money that is more like rent money and less like change. How do other people live with this nothing? I start Googling "chronic pancreatitis disability benefits." Some results are specific to pancreatitis: how it is impossible to secure benefits if you have pancreatitis because you are an alcoholic, and it is because of this very common cause that I suspect pancreatitis is not listed in the Blue Book of accepted conditions and disabilities.[9] The rest of the results are for law practices that specialize in helping people secure benefits. Helping them "win." I could write an entire scholarly monograph on the linguistics of disability benefits within popular culture. Maybe I could write an entire memoir about my attempts at "winning," but I'm not sure yet if winning, in this way, is or should be a part of my living with.

I am also not living with very well right now because I am uncomfortable. What I am with seems like a larger object than what I am living, if that makes sense. But does living with have to mean living with well? People in pain who are addicted to opiates right now are also living with (multiply). I am not living with any better than they are just because I'm not addicted to my medications. And this seems like a fundamental thing to make clear, and then avoid, about living with. It is not about some ideal state. It is not about a hierarchy, either based on the quality of living or on ideas of how some things are easier to live with than others. It is really just a state of mind and this is just a way to describe its biological, linguistic, social, and affective facets. It's to say what it feels like, not how best

9 "Disability Evaluation Under Social Security," *Social Security Administration*, https://www.ssa.gov/disability/professionals/bluebook/AdultListings.htm.

to do it; to imagine multiple bests. While the desire towards open-ness and multiplicity is one I usually find myself moving with, here I am also haunted by what is, perhaps, already the ideal model of living with: Elisabeth Kübler-Ross's five stages towards acceptance. I am not really saying "acceptance." But I'm wary of how it can sound like I am. Living with is a biological fact and physical object that is more complex than coming to terms with and moving through grief over, essentially, this biology. Namely because Kübler-Ross does not really discuss biology. Also because, by outlining a series of five steps that end in an ideal, idealized state (that then gets laid over others who may be grieving or living with, differently, pressuring patients to move rapidly towards a single prescribed end goal), Kübler-Ross's acceptance becomes narrowly defined and universal. Living with does not, necessarily, mean acceptance nor does acceptance always look the way you think it will.

Part of this disavowal, though, is like an adolescent refusal of a parent's suggestion. I can see exactly the way I've moved through Kübler-Ross's pattern. I'm in bargaining now. Denial was the year and a half after I first got sick when I did not stop drinking or make any other changes (though, to be fair, I was not at that point being told that this was permanent). Depression was shortly after, when I did stop drinking and when, given that I was 19 at the time, promptly lost the majority of my friends. Anger is ongoing.

But even so, are these steps really for me, for bodies like mine? On a fundamental level, they presuppose the horribleness, the loss, of what has happened and this is the thing I cannot agree to. It is not all bad. Concurrently, it is not (cannot be for all of us) about this specific form of survivorship. Along with the biological diligence of homeostasis, there is also a state called allostasis: how the body suffers a huge change and adjusts, brings its homeostasis to mainte-nance at different levels.

* * *

Once, I had a fit of anger. Like it fit, around and inside me, well. And is still there, an amorphously bounded object, dissolving while remaining the same, creating an "increasingly subtle fluid."[10] How

10 Gilles Deleuze, "The Fold," trans. Jonathan Strauss, *Yale French Studies*

do you tell two things apart, on levels of visible flesh or molecules? How do you negotiate, especially within a fit of anger, a "perceptual displacement of contours" that is entirely ongoing?[11] I am exactly where one thing ends and another begins, being continually produced by the movement of these two things and sometimes I think it is only my anger that is holding these two things apart. I do just have this thing, in my body, and the thing is pain, and I cannot quite believe that pain is not just a substance like any other.

At a certain point, while reading about the opiate epidemic and pain patients during an ongoing project, I got a question stuck in my head: what's so bad about pain?

This is now incredibly ironic to me, that this was the last sentence I wrote before the day I had to go to the emergency room. Should I read this, now, after, as a joke or as a taunt? As a premonition or an instance of hubris, as if I deserved to be reminded about what's so bad about pain? Or to be reminded how little distance is possible. To be reminded, also really shown for the first time, that so many people around me seem to think the (my) pain is so bad, so why can't I admit it? How do I understand being given intravenous morphine in the emergency room while listening to a woman down the hall being refused anything stronger than ibuprofen? How do I begin to reconcile that the pain really is this bad with also thinking that it is just this thing, in my body, a substance like any other?

But even in experiencing this kind of confusion, it becomes easier, it feels better, to consider pain an object as opposed to a state, a nervous system glitch, or an emotion. Objects are definite. Objects allow for being made of many things simultaneously. Objects are constructed, but also, at a certain point, it no longer always matters why or how. Objects are what they are. Objects can be described. Objects are a thing you can live with. Pain, as an object, becomes substantiated. Pain becomes substantial.

* * *

Another object, also the same one: I have a body made of money. A lot of money, as in many costs, also profit to many other people.

80 (1991): 227–47; 230.
11 Deleuze, "The Fold," 246.

I have a body made of money shaped by the pain I'm in. Right now, I have about $100 worth of prescription drugs in my house. This doesn't seem like a lot, given what it could be. If I didn't have insurance, it would be about $5,000 every month. I do not, right now, make that amount of money, reliably, every year. I don't make that much money because I only work part time, and even at my part time job I frequently leave early, having lost the ability to push through pain and discomfort. If I could work full time, I would make more than twice as much money as I do now at my current hourly rate. This gap, between my potential and actual income, will only grow over time, both in terms of the jobs (and salaries) I will not be qualified for given my work history, and in terms of the savings I will not be able to build. (But then, I think in more morbid moments, how long am I really saving for?) Over time, too, my medical costs will grow. I will need more. More medicine, more medical procedures, eventually. Last year, I was billed upwards of $5,000 by one hospital alone; by a hospital for which my insurance only pays 30% of the cost. I'll need more, generally: ice packs, heating pads, comfortable clothes, food that adheres to a strict diet. None of this is counting the cost of complications. I'll need to try some other objects, too, alternative therapies: acupuncture ($90 per session at the hospital my insurance doesn't pay for), massages (on average, $1/minute). A different, less physically demanding job.

My body made of the money of pain is someone else's profit. Janssen Pharmaceuticals, Bayer, AbbVie, Partners Healthcare, Brigham and Women's Hospital, WestMed Group, CareOne, Johnson & Johnson. So many other companies I am not even aware of purchasing products from (as in: are you buying Tylenol when you buy it or are you meaning to buy a Johnson & Johnson product? Do you know what company owns Johnson & Johnson?) Some of the industries that profit from pain are more apparent than others (who makes the bottles pharmaceuticals come in? The advertisements? The pharmaceutical textbooks?). Or some industries rely more blatantly on advertising than others, or appear more readily to be selling a product than offering relief as such. Like the entire industry devoted to alternative therapies. Without disregarding the effectiveness or helpfulness of such things, like acupuncture, it is still possible to look at the flood of natural supplements, books promising pain relief or improved brain function via special diets and the like and call it what it is: the billion dollar industry of pain, apparent pain, or fear of pain. And how deeply interconnected this industry is to others, like the way that the food industry has capitalized on the growing popularity of gluten-free foods and other health trends to up-market products. Where does the money (or pain) really begin and end? If my pain begins in a specific organ, does it only end when the money of it reaches the pockets of Janssen Pharmaceuticals, the makers of Tramadol (albeit only $2.71 of my $100 per month is spent on this painkiller)? If the money of pain becomes both enormous profit, as in the $35 billion generated by OxyContin for Purdue Pharma since 1995, and perpetuates and newly creates pain (and further expenses, here mainly on the governmental and law enforcement levels), as in the thousands of people currently addicted to or abusing OxyContin, does the object of pain become simply larger or something else altogether?[12]

At least an object is a thing you can live with.

* * *

I know the word is "limitation." If bargaining, I am bargaining for a different definition of this word.

I think about a conversation once with an older woman who has MS, who was telling me about skiing: how she could still do it, despite now being in a wheelchair, but that the process and experience of getting onto and using a monoski was just too much work. Why should she bother? If bargaining, I am bargaining for why I should bother, also for "despite" to be a more recognizably meaningless word than it commonly is.

The thing is, this is not just about living with, for a long time, as if it were just any span of time: it is also inherently about growing up. It can't not be, simply because I've been sick since I was 18. Even though I turned 18 first, got sick a couple months later, the two events are synonymous in retrospect. I had only about two and a half months of disease-free adulthood; it is almost as if I have never

12 Alex Morrell, "The OxyContin Clan: The $14 Billion Newcomer to Forbes 2015 List of Richest U.S. Families," *Forbes,* July 1, 2015, http://www.forbes. com/sites/alexmorrell/2015/07/01/the-oxycontin-clan-the-14-billion-newcomer-to-forbes-2015-list-of-richest-u-s-families/#14cb7821c0e2.

not been a sick adult, never been an adult. Even if turning 18, getting sick, had been more temporally spread out, there are only so many points in time you can look to or across at that age, mostly ahead.

I am and am not a young woman. I am and am not also an old woman.

Having much more to look ahead to than back at, at 18, I think of the passage in Claudia Rankine's *Don't Let Me Be Lonely*, about westerns: "Just before he dies he says, I am not going to make it. Where? Not going to make it where? On some level, maybe, the phrase simply means not going to make it into the next day, hour, minute or perhaps the next second.... On another level always implicit is the sense that it means he is not going to make it to his own death. Perhaps in the back of all of our minds is the life expectancy for our generation."[13]

Is my generation people who are my age now, people who have had chronic pancreatitis as long as I have, people who are 48, people who have the same prognosis or live in the same mortality rates? What is the difference between a generation and a peer? Are my peers the people who peer-reviewed my first book, written mostly when I was twenty, who wrote in their reviews as if, assuredly, I must be an older person with a PhD who is also a man?

This is why I had bought a book called *Life Disrupted: Getting Real About Chronic Illness in Your Twenties and Thirties* after the conversation about diligence.[14] Being sick, young, is not like being sick at other ages, ages at which it may be more normal, have become more regular among one's peers, to be sick. Nor, though, is it at all like being a pediatric patient.

I think about growing up, and growing into, and growing out of, and growing pains.

* * *

I had started to read books about aging, but they weren't entirely helpful. Or I just wasn't paying attention. What I failed to notice,

---

13 Claudia Rankine, *Don't Let Me Be Lonely: An American Lyric* (Saint Paul, MN: Graywolf Press, 2004), 24.
14 Laurie Edwards, *Life Disrupted: Getting Real About Chronic Illness in Your Twenties and Thirties* (New York: Walker Books, 2011).

and what is now astonishingly obvious: where are all the people growing up sick? Not just the normal aging-related conditions, the mid-life crises and terminal illnesses, the childhood illnesses. Where are the sick 20-year-olds? The sick emerging adults? The sick kids who became sick adults and not only the sick kids who stayed that way, who died as kids or became completely better before becoming an adult. As if this, a becoming completely better, was the only way they could become an adult. A prerequisite for adulthood.

As if one cannot conceive of an adult who is not able.

Because sick kids staying sick is too sad? Because no one wants no future? Because staying sick is the opposite of growing up? Because 23 is not supposed to be middle-aged? But, then, what's so special about middle age that it should be reserved only for the not sick?

And then, you think, okay: maybe there are just not that many 20-year-olds writing memoirs. But even this does not explain the vast majority of memoirs that do exist: memoirs about what it was like to have a sick child, to lose one, or to *have been* one; all narratives beginning and ending with Tiny Tim and all other characters who had to die within their stories because it was inconceivable that they may, how it may have even been possible, for them to continue living as they were.

Even as the archetype, Tiny Tim is also something of an exception. Because given industrial revolution-era Britain, he really could not have lived longer (in terms of medical knowledge and technology, and attitudes therein). Which actually puts the lack of portrayals of sick young adults, now, in an even more questionable or illegitimate position, because given the state of medicine, so many diseases that had been deadly are not now: more and more young people will be living with longer and longer. Where are they?

I think about growing into, and growing pains. And growing up, as a form of reaching.

And what is and is not reachable and what cannot, will not, be reached and what cannot be reached out of.

Because sick kids staying sick is too sad? Because growing, in its very definition, denies the possibility of a low, that reaching a low can be a part of growing? How last week, at my doctor's, my blood tests were the worst they've been in years. And, of course, you think: this is the *been spreading*. And why am I still surprised to see the numbers? Because my doctor had been optimistic? Which

I believed; this was not the doctor who told me he would not, and then did, find the adenoma. Because, even knowing otherwise, I still thought I had just been growing up, how everything is supposed to get better when you get older, so much more freedom, how you can do everything you want, not how your organs cannot do everything, how growing is more and more and is not, ever, more of a bad thing. An incompatible yet simultaneous increase and decrease; a flat plane.

* * *

Taking growing up for granted, taking for granted its being only an increase of good things, seems possible and embedded mostly because this is not the 1800s or earlier. Historically, "nearly 60 percent of deaths happened to people 15 or younger and another 20 percent to those between 15 and 45."[15] The fact of growing up, now, is not entirely a matter of human biology, given that the life span in the 1800s was 70, comparable to the 76 years it is today. It's just that the life expectancies were so different then, approximately 38 and 36 for men and women, respectively. You just had to make it past that to live a long time.

Being able to grow up, how this happened over time, may not have been entirely a matter of human biology, but it was definitely a matter of biology, of science and medicine. Also money. And industrial development, public health campaigns, safer birth procedures, antibiotics, urbanism. All matters of being able to get people past a certain point and expectation.

The expectation became farther and farther away.

Not that such a point has ever been a constant, or ultimately based on anything other than a social and historical construct: adulthood.

Being a social and historical construct it would be, on the one hand, easy to detail the specifics of these constructs through time and across medical, biological, legal, and social realms. On the other hand, this would quickly become complicated and only serve to

15 Meghan Daum, "The Prime of Life by Steven Mintz," *The New York Times,* June 15, 2015, http://www.nytimes.com/2015/06/21/books/review/the-prime-of-life-by-steven-mintz.html.

diffuse the beliefs underlying this construct such that they become unrecognizable.

It would be simpler to define adulthood through its negative, in the sense of its reverse image. An adult is not someone, a person and a body, who has to have pediatric-sized equipment used during surgeries; who has a pediatric-sized body (quite literally; I am basically the same weight now, at 23, I was when I was 13) because of weight-loss in illness; who cannot hold a full-time job; who has not reached financial independence; who lacks a freedom of movement (how do you move away from the doctors you have to see every few months? How do you travel if, on a daily basis, you can barely eat most foods and, in the event of unforeseen circumstances, can become seriously ill?); who cannot fully exercise rights in relation to substances (I am of drinking age, but did you know that pancreatitis patients who continue to drink are significantly more likely to die within 10 years?); an adult is not someone who, yesterday, had a stranger say that they looked fragile, who had not yet realized that fragility was an accepted visual marker of adult ablebodiedness. And if adulthood is a social construct than does it truly matter what my chronological age is if all of the above are also true, if I am consistently unable to fully access the social nature of adulthood and its concurrent freedoms? "Freedom is a boundary concept that delimits the realm of all other objects we can know."[16] We know adulthood as, through, and by its freedom. We know freedom as adulthood, especially in youth: freedom is the imagined area beyond what we can know is coming next.

* * *

I know the word is limitation. I know I do not feel free.

I do not feel free, and the following are some preliminary reasons: One, that the object of adulthood is freedom. Two, that the freedom of adulthood is defined by rights dependent on age. Three, being unable to fully exercise these rights is being unable to be an adult, ultimately regardless of chronological age.

16 Corinne Field, *The Struggle for Equal Adulthood: Gender, Race, Age, and the Fight for Citizenship in Antebellum America* (Chapel Hill, NC: University of North Carolina Press, 2014), 5.

Four, that it is inconceivable to be an adult who is not able because of the way that sickness and disability prevent the exercise of certain rights but also because of fundamental and embedded beliefs about ablebodiedness, health and growth. These beliefs are seen especially within psychology, and via the way that psychology and therapeutic narratives have become pervasive within popular conceptions of selfhood and particularly adult selfhood. To quote Abraham Maslow, an influential psychologist in the 1960s, "[I]n practically every human being, and certainly in almost every newborn baby, that there is an active will towards health, an impulse toward growth, or toward the actualization of human potentialities."[17] Growth and health are synonymous. And you cannot grow on a flat plane.

* * *

Months ago, I cried because of how much I want. I said exactly this, to my partner, while crying. And across so many drafts of this piece, it has always started with this sentence, about all of the things I want in my life, how I imagine them in and with my body, or apart from them. I know the word is limitation, and I am beginning to know or feel that what will come to be most limited is what I want and what I am able to have; that because of this tension between desire and freedom, I will and maybe mostly will not feel free. It is this feeling of not feeling free that will be the hardest to live with. It almost doesn't matter about the specifics of my body, it doesn't really matter that I can't go out every weekend or eat whatever I want. Those things are what diligence is for. But what form of diligence is capable of reshaping the flat plane of limitations, the way it flattens (across) a sense of freedom? I am not saying that I am not, at the same time, also extremely privileged. Both can be true. I am really just saying that this is not about (only) that kind of material freedom or privilege.

17 Eva Illouz, *Saving the Modern Soul: Therapy, Emotions, and the Culture of Self-Help* (Berkeley, CA: University of California Press, 2008), 159.

Because maybe a sense of freedom and especially one supported by rights pertaining to the exercise of desire is really just about concealing death.

How maybe feeling free is just the feeling of not dying, and maybe the freedom of adulthood and what makes the synonymy of growth and health absolutely necessary for maintaining this freedom is that it produces an ability to conceive of a self who is growing, growing up, getting better, and not only always already growing towards death.

The illusion, work and feeling of this can be difficult to maintain.

The impossibility and, therefore, drastic reimagining that becomes necessary of the relationship between freedom and adulthood is a fundamental aspect of the experience of being sick young and growing up sick.

* * *

I have wondered about the "getting real" in the subtitle of *Life Disrupted*. Getting real about what? How do you acquire realness? If this is something you had to get, what was it you had before?

I remain attached to a fantasy of middle-age.

In some ways, the fantasy is a joke, made up of the gaps created by overlaying a figure of middle age onto my body, how they do and do not align. In this way, as per my previous comments about statistics, it is really a joke about systemic sexism. Underlying the joke, though, is an antagonism against "getting real." This is not acceptance.

* * *

While doing research for a project about the opiate epidemic, I got a phrase stuck in my head: the idea of getting addicted to thinking about your body in the future, or to thinking about your body in a different future. The reasoning behind this idea is loosely based on the physiology of opiates, and their role in producing placebo effects, and the fact that it is ultimately a person's expectations of pain relief, expectations about what is about to happen, that are responsible for releasing endogenous and pain relieving opiates within a body. Of course, all of these points are more complicated than this. But it is still interesting and possible to imagine a body capable of becoming addicted to the pain relief produced by being able to imagine that body in a (different) future. Because what such a model entails is the importance and function of temporally specific imaginings and the both direct and looping relationship between what is imagined and the biology involved. "Addiction" is figured as the threat of releasing, too far, into this cycle but, still — why *not* middle age, within this?

"The hope is that the labor of maintaining optimism will not be negated by the work of world-maintenance as such and will allow the flirtation with *some* good-life sweetness to continue."[18]

Also while reading for and about the opiate epidemic, I came across a Marxist conception of a "freedom with." In short, a conception of freedom opposed to commonly neoliberal freedoms that are formulated as "freedom from" (from other people, from encroaching institutions) in that Marx figures the atomistic nature of a "freedom from" as inherently anti-free; "freedom with" entails always, only, a freedom as freedom *with* others.[19] A freedom suited to always already *living with*.

And what about internally? If there is no "freedom from" externally,[20] why should it be assumed that one would be possible internally, as if one could be free from encroaching physicality? And when it isn't, why wouldn't a "freedom with" be the positive possibility?

I mean, I know the word is "limitation." I know this will be work, more and more work. But I also feel it's possible to follow the contours of a fold, follow it into an "increasingly subtle fluid," where, maybe, everything (some things) are both more fluid and subtler

18 Lauren Berlant, "Slow Death (Sovereignty, Obesity, Lateral Agency)," *Critical Inquiry* 33.4 (2011): 754–80.
19 Wendy Brown, *States of Injury: Power and Freedom in Late Modernity* (Princeton, NJ: Princeton University Press, 1995) and "Learning to Love Again: An Interview with Wendy Brown," *Contretemps* 6 (2006): 25–42.
20 Inasmuch as what is initially figured as a "freedom from" — the freedom to not have to purchase health insurance as governmentally mandated, say, as a freedom from regulation — often becomes something distinctly un-free, as in the millions of people who may soon find themselves unable to access healthcare and who, in short, may die sooner.

in both directions. How can I move along this fold or any without retaining a "middle age"?

If this will be a *freedom with,* it should be a freedom with fantasy as much as with biology.

For years, what was difficult was not knowing exactly what was wrong with me. I had gotten sick so suddenly, so acutely, that when it was over it seemed actually over. No one was telling me that it would become chronic. No one was telling me, either, exactly why this had just happened. There was no diagnosis. And this confusion and lack of information came to fit with an increasingly synonymous lack of information within critical theory and disability studies: where were all the bodies like mine? The synonymy of these confusions made writing *Ghostbodies,* my book detailing this very lack of narratives within theory, relatively easy to write. Now, though, I know exactly what's wrong with me, even if I do not know exactly why; the why is no longer something I am concerned about. This is not a diagnostic confusion, but a prognostic confusion. For the past year, since last fall when I did finally receive a definitive diagnosis, I have started projects over and over. Some I've finished, mostly I have felt unfinished. This confusion does not fit well with anything else. It is difficult to give form to. And in a way, this actually makes perfect sense: when you do not know what is coming next, when there is a future but what it is is deeply unclear, what else is there to do but start over and over? And yet this, now, does feel finished. This feels like both a love letter and a goodbye. Throughout not only this text but *Ghostbodies* and every other project I've started and left this year, the urgency of my questions has been focused in two main directions: how can or will I live "in theory," and how can and will I live "in life"? In theory, I demand rights to make up for what has been lacking. In life, I work and I imagine. In theory, I love what has been found, the idea of what will be found, and the very ability to make coherent demands that can be answered. In life, is this enough? "What should I be cured of? To find what condition, what life?"[21] In theory, I can demand and I can demonstrate and I can be sick all I want but, in life, is this enough? How far can theory extend? In living with, within the form of a visceralized body, a body that is deeply imaginative, a body that is deeply open (to

21 Roland Barthes, *Mourning Diary* (New York: Hill & Wang, 2010), 97.

others), should it not be time to fully turn towards those others? How far can we extend this, together; live with, together?

* * *

How do you live with something for a long time? All of the time, I imagine.

Bibliography

Akil, M., R.S. Amos, and P. Stewart. "Infertility May Sometimes be Associated with NSAID Consumption." *Rhueumatolgy* 35.1 (1996): 76–78. Doi: 10.1093/rheumatology/35.1.76.

Alexander, Christopher, Sara Ishikawa, Murray Silverstein, Max Jacobson, Ingrid Fiksdahl-King, and Shlomo Angel. *A Pattern Language: Towns, Buildings, Construction.* New York: Oxford University Press, 1977.

Alexander, Elizabeth. *The Light of the World: A Memoir.* New York: Grand Central Publishing, 2015.

American Chronic Pain Association. "The Art of Pain Management." http://theacpa.org/uploads/Art_and_Music_final.pdf.

Andrey Smith, Peter. "Can the Bacteria in Your Gut Explain Your Mood?" *The New York Times Magazine,* June 23, 2015, http://www.nytimes.com/2015/06/28/magazine/can-the-bacteria-in-your-gut-explain-your-mood.html.

Aubrey, Allison. "Prozac in the Yogurt Aisle: Can 'Good' Bacteria Chill Us Out?" *National Public Radio,* July 14, 2015, http://www.npr.org/sections/thesalt/2015/07/14/422623067/prozac-in-the-yogurt-aisle-can-good-bacteria-chill-us-out.

Barthes, Roland. *Mourning Diary.* New York: Hill & Wang, 2010.

Beilock, Sian. *How the Body Knows its Mind: The Surprising Power of the Physical Environment to Influence How You Think and Feel.* New York: Atria Books, 2015.

Bending, Lucy. "Approximation, Suggestion and Analogy: Translating Pain Into Language." *The Yearbook of English Studies* 36.1 (2006): 131–37.

Berfield, Susan, Jef Feeley, and Margaret Cronin Fisk. "Johnson & Johnson Has a Baby Powder Problem," *Bloomberg Business Week,* March 31, 2016, http://www.bloomberg.com/features/

2016-baby-powder-cancer-lawsuits/.

Berlant, Lauren. *Cruel Optimism*. Durham, NC: Duke University Press, 2007.

———. "Slow Death (Sovereignty, Obesity, Lateral Agency)." *Critical Inquiry* 33.4 (2011): 754–80.

Birke, Lynda. *Feminism and the Biological Body*. New Brunswick, NJ: Rutgers University Press, 2000.

Boyer, Anne. "Not Writing." *The Poetry Foundation,* 2015, https://www.poetryfoundation.org/poems-and-poets/poems/detail/58316.

Braidotti, Rosi. "Enduring Self-Health." *Science as Culture* 7.3 (1998): 423–29.

Breckenridge, C. and Candace Vogler. "The Critical Limits of Embodiment: Disability's Criticism." *Public Culture* 13.3 (2001): 349–57.

Brown, Wendy. *States of Injury: Power and Freedom in Late Modernity*. Princeton, NJ: Princeton University Press, 1995.

———. "Learning to Love Again: An Interview with Wendy Brown." *Contretemps* 6 (2006): 25–42.

Cairns, Stephen and Jane Jacobs. *Buildings Must Die: A Perverse View of Architecture*. Cambridge, MA: MIT Press, 2014.

Charmaz, Kathy. *Good Days, Bad Days: The Self and Chronic Illness in Time*. New Brunswick, NJ: Rutgers University Press, 1993.

Clare, Eli. "Stolen Bodies, Reclaimed Bodies: Disability and Queerness." *Public Culture* 13.3 (2001): 359–65.

Cvetkovich, Ann. *Depression: A Public Feeling*. Durham, NC: Duke University Press, 2012.

Damasio, Antonio, *The Feeling of What Happens: Body and Emotion in the Making of Consciousness*. New York: Mariner Books, 1999.

———. *Looking for Spinoza: Joy, Sorrow, and the Feeling Brain*. San Diego, CA: Harcourt, 2003.

Daum, Meghan. "The Prime of Life by Steven Mintz." *The New York Times,* June 15, 2015, http://www.nytimes.com/2015/06/21/books/review/the-prime-of-life-by-steven-mintz.html.

Davis, Allison. "For Man With Cystic Fibrosis, Death is Like a Deadline." *National Public Radio,* May 1, 2015, http://www.npr.org/2015/05/01/403303311/for-man-with-cystic-fibrosis-death-is-like-a-deadline.

De Botton, Alain. *The Pleasures and Sorrows of Work*. New York: Pantheon Books, 2009.

Deleuze, Gilles. "The Fold," translated by Jonathan Strauss. *Yale French Studies* 80 (1991): 227–47.

Dickinson, Emily. *The Complete Poems of Emily Dickinson*. Boston, MA: Little, Brown, 1924.

Dolphin-Krute, Maia. *Ghostbodies: Towards a New Theory of Invalidism*. Bristol, UK: Intellect, 2017.

Edwards, Laurie. *Life Disrupted: Getting Real About Chronic Illness in Your Twenties and Thirties*. New York: Walker Books, 2011.

Eagleton, Terry. "It is not quite true that I have a body and not quite true that I am one either." *London Review of Books,* July 22, 1993, http://www.lrb.co.uk/v15/n10/terry-eagleton/it-is-not-quite-true-that-i-have-a-body-and-not-quite-true-that-i-am-one-either.

Emblem Health. "Who's Caring for You?" http://blog.emblem-health.com/.

Field, Corinne. *The Struggle for Equal Adulthood: Gender, Race, Age, and the Fight for Citizenship in Antebellum America*. Chapel Hill, NC: University of North Carolina Press, 2014.

Foucault, Michel. *The Birth of the Clinic: An Archaeology of Medical Perception,* translated by Alan Sheridan Smith. New York: Pantheon Books, 1973.

———. "Madness, the Absence of Work," translated by Peter Stastny and Deniz Sengel. *Critical Inquiry* 21.2 (1995): 290–98.

Frank, Adam and Elizabeth Wilson. "Like Minded." *Critical Inquiry* 38.4 (2012): 870–77.

Gallagher, Shaun. *How the Body Shapes the Mind*. Oxford, UK: Oxford University Press, 2005.

Graeber, David. *The Utopia of Rules: On Technology, Stupidity, and the Secret Joys of Bureaucracy*. Brooklyn, NY: Melville House Press, 2015.

Gulli, Cathy. "The Brain-Gut Connection." *MacLean's* 121.45 (2008): 64–67.

Hall, Donald. *Life Work*. Boston, MA: Beacon Press, 1993.

Hardt, Michael and Antonio Negri. *Declaration*. New York: Argo-Navis, 2012.

Harper, Carly and Ingrid Richardson. "Imaging the Visceral Soma: A Corporeal Feminist Interpretation." *Indo-Pacific Journal of Phenomenology* 6.3 (2006): 1–13.

Safe. Dir. Todd Haynes. Los Angeles: Sony Pictures Classic, 1995. DVD.

Healy, Beth and Todd Wallack. "Madoff Client to Return $625 Million." *The Boston Globe,* December 8, 2010, http://archive. boston.com/yourtown/boston/roxbury/articles/2010/12/08/ madoff_client_settles_with_us_for_625m/.

Hunter, Ian. "The History of Theory." *Critical Inquiry* 33.1 (2006): 78–112.

Hussain, Zareena. "MIT to Pay Victims $1.85 Million in Fernald Radiation Settlement." *The Tech,* January 7, 1998, http://tech. mit.edu/V117/N65/bfernald.65n.html.

Illouz, Eva. *Saving the Modern Soul: Therapy, Emotions, and the Culture of Self-Help.* Berkeley, CA: University of California Press, 2008.

"Joel E. Smilow: Executive Profile." *Bloomberg.com,* 2017, http:// www.bloomberg.com/ research/stocks/private/person.asp?pers onId=4141786&privcapId=10947511.

Kabat Zinn, Jon. "In Touch With Your Skin." *Mindfulness* 4.4 (2013): 392–93.

Kafer, Alison. *Feminist, Queer, Crip.* Bloomington, IN: Indiana University Press, 2013.

Kirby, Vicki and Elizabeth Wilson. "Feminist Conversations with Vicki Kirby and Elizabeth A. Wilson." *Feminist Theory* 12.2 (2011): 227–34.

Kramer, Peter. *Listening to Prozac: The Landmark Book about Antidepressants and the Remaking of the Self.* New York: Penguin Books, 1997.

Kristeva, Julia. *The Powers of Horror: An Essay on Abjection,* translated by Leon Roudiez. New York: Columbia University Press, 1982.

———. "A Tragedy and A Dream: Disability Revisited." *Irish Theological Quarterly* 78.3 (2013): 219–30.

Latour, Bruno. "Why Has Critique Run Out of Steam? From Matters of Fact to Matters of Concern." *Critical Inquiry* 30.2 (2004): 225–48.

Leder, Drew. *The Absent Body*. Chicago, IL: University of Chicago Press, 1990.

———. "Flesh and Blood: A Proposed Supplement to Merleau-Ponty." *Human Studies* 13.3 (1990): 209–19.

Lochlann Jain, Sarah. "Living in Prognosis: Toward an Elegiac Politics." *Representations* 98.1 (2007): 77–92.

———. *Malignant: How Cancer Becomes Us*. Berkeley, CA: University of California Press, 2013.

Malabou, Catherine. *Ontology of the Accident: An Essay on Destructive Plasticity*. Cambridge, UK: Polity, 2012.

Manguso, Sarah. *Ongoingness: The End of a Diary*. Minneapolis, MN: Graywolf Press, 2015.

McRuer, Robert. *Crip Theory: Cultural Signs of Queerness and Disability*. New York: New York University Press, 2006.

Mitchell, David. "Body Solitaire: The Singular Subject of Disability Autobiography." *American Quarterly* 52.2 (2000): 311–15.

Morrell, Alex. "The OxyContin Clan: The $14 Billion Newcomer to Forbes 2015 List of Richest U.S. Families." *Forbes,* July 1, 2015, http://www.forbes.com/sites/alexmorrell/2015/07/01/the-oxy-contin-clan-the-14-billion-newcomer-to-forbes-2015-list-of-rich-est-u-s-families/.

Nasar, Sylvia. "Richard Nessen, 66, Ex-President of Teaching Hospital in Boston." *The New York Times,* October 23, 1998, http://www.nytimes.com/1998/10/23/business/richard-nesson-66-ex-president-of-teaching-hospital-in-boston.html.

Nussbaum, Emily. "Candy Girl." *The New Yorker,* March 30, 2015, http://www.newyorker.com/ magazine/2015/03/30/candy-girl.

Porter, James. "[The Body in Theory]." *Public Culture* 11.3 (1990): 440–42.

Puar, Jasbir K. "Prognosis Time: Towards a Geopolitics of Affect, Debility and Capacity." *Women & Performance: a journal of feminist theory* 19.2 (2009): 161–72.

Ralph, Michael. "Flirt[ing] With Death But 'Still Alive': The Sexual Dimensions of Surplus Time in Hip Hop Fantasy." *Cultural Dynamics* 18.1 (2006): 61–88.

Ramachandran, V.S. "Consciousness and Body Image: Lessons from Phantom Limbs, Capgras Syndrome and Pain Asymbolia." *Philosophical Transactions of the Royal Society B: Biological Sciences* 353 (1998): 1851–59.

Rankine, Claudia. *Don't Let Me Be Lonely: An American Lyric.* Saint Paul, MN: Graywolf Press, 2004.

Sacks, Oliver. "Witty Ticcy Ray." *London Review of Books,* March 19, 1981, 3–5, http://www.lrb.co.uk/vo3/no5/oliver-sacks/witty-ticcy-ray.

———. "The Leg." *London Review of Books,* June 17, 1982, 3–5, http://www.lrb.co.uk/ vo4/n11/oliver-sacks/the-leg.

Simic, Charles. *The Monster Loves His Labyrinth: Notebooks.* New York: Ausable Press, 2008.

Shakespeare, William. "Sonnet 146." *Poets.org,* https://www.poets.org/poetsorg/poem/poor-soul-centre-my-sinful-earth-sonnet-146.

Solomon, Andrew. "The Anatomy of Melancholy." *The New Yorker,* January 12, 1998, http://www.newyorker.com/magazine/1998/01/12/anatomy-of-melancholy.

Sontag, Susan. *Illness as Metaphor and AIDS and its Metaphors.* New York: Farrar, Straus and Giroux, 1978.

Stone, S., et. al. "Non-Steroidal Anti-Inflammatory Drugs and Reversible Infertility." *Drug Safety* 25.8 (2002): 545–51.

Sutherland, Stephani. "Pain That Won't Quit." *Scientific American,* December 2014, http://www.erythromelalgia.org/Portals/0/ProspectsforTreatingChronicPainScientificAmerican.pdf.

Weisz, George. *Chronic Disease in the 20th Century: A History.* Baltimore, MD: Johns Hopkins University Press, 2014.

Wilson, Elizabeth A. "Gut Feminism." *differences: A Journal of Feminist Cultural Studies* 15.3 (2004): 66–94.

———. "The Work of Antidepressants: Preliminary Notes on How to Build an Alliance Between Feminism and Psychopharmacology." *BioSocieties* 1 (2006): 125–31.

———. *Psychosomatic: Feminism and the Neurological Body.* Durham, NC: Duke University Press, 2015.

Zambreno, Kate. "Melancholy and the Infinite Sadness." *The New Inquiry,* February 28, 2013, http://thenewinquiry.com/essays/melancholy-and-the-infinite-sadness/.

"The local mechanisms of mind . . . are not all in the head.

Cognition leaks out into body and world."

— Andy Clark, *Supersizing the Mind*

brainstorm books

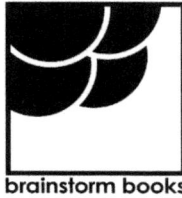

Current developments in psychoanalysis, psychology, philosophy, and cognitive and neuroscience confirm the profound importance of expression and interpretation in forming the mind's re-workings of its intersubjective, historical and planetary environments. Brainstorm Books seeks to publish cross-disciplinary work on the becomings of the extended and enactivist mind, especially as afforded by semiotic experience. Attending to the centrality of expression and impression to living process and to the ecologically-embedded situatedness of mind is at the heart of our enterprise. We seek to cultivate and curate writing that attends to the ways in which art and aesthetics are bound to, and enhance, our bodily, affective, cognitive, developmental, intersubjective, and transpersonal practices.

Brainstorm Books is an imprint of the "Literature and the Mind" group at the University of California, Santa Barbara, a research and teaching concentration hosted within the Department of English and supported by affiliated faculty in Comparative Literature, Religious Studies, History, the Life Sciences, Psychology, Cognitive Science, and the Arts.

http://mind.english.ucsb.edu/brainstorm-books/

www.ingramcontent.com/pod-product-compliance
Lightning Source LLC
Chambersburg PA
CBHW071556200326
41519CB00021BB/6779